MW01247080

Diagnosed

Diagnosed

Inspirational Stories After an
Alarming Medical Diagnosis

MARK AND MARY KAY LISTON

XULON ELITE

Xulon Press Elite
2301 Lucien Way #415
Maitland, FL 32751
407.339.4217
www.xulonpress.com

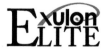

Paperback ISBN-13: 978-1-66287-924-1
Hard Cover ISBN-13: 978-1-66287-925-8
Ebook ISBN-13: 978-1-66287-926-5

Endorsements

After literally nudging Mark Liston, for years, to write a book filled with his "OMG" Blogs – (each blog better that the last) he finally produces a personal story of love, faith, and hope.

"Diagnosed: Inspirational Stories After an Alarming Medical Diagnosis" is a compelling book filled with 26 powerful stories of individuals who have faced a diagnosis head-on and emerged stronger on the other side – followed by Mark's personal journey after he was diagnosed with lung cancer.

Through these inspiring journeys, readers are given a glimpse of hope, courage, and resilience in the face of adversity.

I am one of these stories – shared with an enormous amount of pride, and the hope it helps many. Covid 19 saved my life. Sounds ODD? But it did. My story is Case #10 - Were it not for Covid, I may not be here. I'm not alone....this book and all the 26 stories, is a must-read for anyone who needs a reminder that there is light at the end of the tunnel, no matter what life throws their way."

Nancy Friedman
Founder – Chairman of Telephone Doctor
Telephone Doctor Customer Service Training
Author . Speaker . Corporate Training

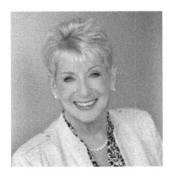

Faith is such a steadfast friend when time becomes precious to the point of running out. But God is great all the time for those who receive Him as Mark and MK know so well.

They are one of the most faith-filled couples I know, and that faith and inspiration shines through in this powerful collection of stories that readers are sure to embrace.

I lost a father much too soon to a sudden heart attack. I've also hung on to every precious moment with a mother whose dementia takes a little piece of her away every single day. Be it fast or slow, God is in charge and each day is a gift. Thank you for this wonderful book and the important reminder to embrace that gift to the fullest.

Dina Dwyer-Owens
Author, Speaker, Franchise Leader, IFA Hall of Fame
Former Chair and CEO Neighborly

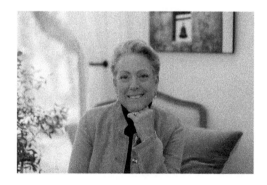

CONTENTS

INTRO

This book contains stories about people who received a life-altering diagnosis. Most are stories of survival and healing. A couple stories included are about people who didn't survive. One is my brother-in-law. The other was my best friend for years.

We are retired now. For years we've threatened to author a book. Mark is the writer and Mary Kay is the editor. We just needed a sign, an inspiration. It happened on November 3, 2022, when a doctor told us, "I'm sorry. Looks like you have lung cancer, Mark."

Mark never smoked. His dad died 55 years ago. He was a heavy Camel smoker, but Mark hadn't been around secondhand smoke since then. Mark was only thirteen when he died.

For the next 76 days Mark chronicled every day. Every thought. Every doctor's appointment, hospital appointment, and new medicine. As the 76 days were winding down, he woke up one morning thinking, "I'm missing it!"

We realized that morning that the real focus of this book should be those who had faced similar issues.

That day, January 11, 2023, Mark posted this on Facebook:

> *I've been drafting a book for the last two months and am to the point where I want to interview others who have faced cancer or other life-threatening challenges . . . or have a close relative who've faced this. The book is about having patience, going through the process of working with doctors, and providing support. If you would like me to include your story, please send me a private message on Facebook. Thanks.*

The response from friends, former high school classmates, and people we worked with in the past was overwhelming. Each survived cancer or another life-altering illness or was a caretaker for someone who had. Each one offered unique insights.

Ninety percent of those interviewed shared the importance their faith in God and in prayer played in their story.

Since Mark was five years old and his parents sent him to St. Paul Lutheran School, he always had had a faith in Jesus and in prayer. Mary Kay was raised in the church, as well.

Tim Tebow

Remember how Tim Tebow was ridiculed on social media for taking a knee in the end zone after a touchdown? Canadian broadcaster Don Cherry (among others) wrote that former Denver Broncos quarterback Tim Tebow, a devout Christian, was mocked by the media for taking a knee to pray after scoring a touchdown in his breakout rookie season in 2010. He wrote, "The late-night leftie talk shows made fun of Tim, to the cartoonists in the paper he was a joke and they made fun of him."

They called it "Tebowing."

Joseph Kennedy

Compare Tebow's experience to that of Joseph Kennedy. Here is how ABC News reported it:

> A former public high school football coach in Washington state who famously lost his job for leading prayers on the field after games will be reinstated by the spring of next year, court documents show.
>
> A joint stipulation filed in Washington state district court on Tuesday by attorneys representing Joseph Kennedy and lawyers for Bremerton School District stated that "Kennedy is

to be reinstated to his previous position as assistant coach of the Bremerton High School football team on or before March 15, 2023."

Kennedy's attorney, Jeremy Dys, confirmed to ABC News that the coach will be moving back to Bremerton, Washington, from Florida later this year to return to his part-time job with the team. It's expected he'd take the field again for the fall 2023 football season.

Damar Hamlin

And how about Damar Hamlin? Here is how the New York Times reported:

As the ambulance carrying the injured Buffalo Bills player Damar Hamlin rolled slowly off the field in Cincinnati Monday night, a huddle of players and team staff knelt in a massive yet intimate circle on the field. They bowed their heads, some placing hands on each other's shoulders and others with tears streaming down their faces, in a moment of spontaneous prayer led by the team's chaplain, Len Vanden Bos. The hushed crowd at Paycor Stadium burst into applause as the players knelt and again as they rose.

It was the first of many prayers in an extraordinary display of public piety that unfurled across the country in the hours and days after Mr. Hamlin's collapse, after what looked like a routine collision early in the game. Mr. Hamlin suffered cardiac arrest on the field and was in critical condition on Wednesday night at the University of Cincinnati Medical Center.

"Please pray for our brother," the Bills' quarterback, Josh Allen, wrote on Twitter, where players and coaches across the league

shared similar messages. All 32 N.F.L. teams changed their Twitter profile pictures to a message reading "PRAY FOR DAMAR," in the style of Mr. Hamlin's blue jersey. Fans huddled in vigils outside the hospital in Cincinnati and outside Highmark Stadium in Buffalo, where Jill Kelly, the wife of former Bills quarterback Jim Kelly, led a crowd in prayer.

The Difference

What was the difference between the three situations?

Why would the same people who ridiculed Tebow and Kennedy be supporting the prayers for Hamlin? I have no idea. Because of Hamlin's injury compared to the other two situations not involving an injury? Perhaps.

It was because when a person is put in a life-threatening situation, life and death come intensely into focus. It might be that when faced with death, a concern wells up in most every human: what will happen to me when the doctors close my eyes for the final time?

What you are going to see in this book are stories of people for whom prayer is a part of their lives.

When the doctor told me, "I'm sorry—it looks like you have lung cancer" my prayers didn't change. Mine were simply, "Thy will be done" from the Lord's Prayer.

At one point, years ago, the big C, *cancer*, and heart disease were death sentences. It isn't any longer.

You'll also read that having the right attitude can have an influence on every aspect of your life.

I hope these stories–along with the 76 days of my own story–inspire you. Enjoy. Learn. Change.

Medical News Today reports that one in two women and one in three men will have cancer at one point of their lifetime.

This book prepares you for those you know, or the person you see in the mirror today, should you face such a challenge.

Mark wrote this in the first person. Mary Kay has had as much to do with this as he did. We are partners in life, partners in love, partners in this book. Every word he wrote she edited. And changed. And fixed. And made it much better for you!

Thank God we became, as Ephesians 5:31 reads, "one flesh."

This book is divided into two sections. The first section is Diagnosis stories from over twenty-five people. They cover a wide variety of cancer diagnoses.

The second section is the 76 days of my personal diagnosis of lung cancer. My goal was to share what it is like getting a diagnosis, on a day-by-day basis – until we knew that I was in the clear and no more worries about this initial diagnosis.

Also included will be pictures of many mentioned in the book.

We pray this will bring God's blessing to you.

Mark and Mary Kay Liston

Case #1:

Heather - Breast Cancer & Double Mastectomy

This interview was so special for me. MK and I worked with Heather. She was the corporate controller of our company when she got breast cancer. All of us quickly knew all about it. What I didn't know was her entire story.

This is another example of what women with breast cancer can elect to do. Most importantly, as you will read, it is the attitude that you can take and what her belief in God did for her.

Heather was busy! An important job with our company, two kids (eleven and eight) who both made select sports teams and were on ballfields all summer. Outside of work, Heather spent her weekends either watching kids play or working in the concession stand helping to raise money for the teams.

One day in January 2013 Heather's husband, Jeffrey, noticed a lump in Heather's breast. He mentioned it to her, and she decided to be proactive and called her primary care physician (PCP) the next day. The lump wasn't that big, but the PCP thought it was worthy of a mammogram. The mammogram showed that there was something there.

Within a week and a half, Heather went from not noticing anything to having a biopsy.

Since they moved to Waco years before, Heather and Jeffrey had become friends with their PCP. When Heather got the call to go to the PCP's office the next day, she wasn't concerned.

The two of them soon heard, "I'm sorry to tell you this but it is breast cancer."

The doctor asked if she had any questions, and Heather responded, "I give blood every eight weeks and I just donated recently. Can this be passed on through my blood to anyone else?"

No surprise to me that her first question would be about others, not herself.

She did not tell anyone at work at first. She was still trying to digest those words that had made her breathless. Sure, she could stay busy with her responsibilities at work, but when her head hit the pillow, there was nothing else on her mind.

The next month or so was a whirlwind. Within two weeks they met with an oncologist and a surgeon. She and her husband needed to make decisions regarding what would happen next and treatments: lumpectomy, mastectomy, double mastectomy? All she wanted was for the doctor to tell her what she needed to do next.

Heather decided to take the BRCA gene test. If she carried that gene, doctors would recommend a hysterectomy because it increases the chances for ovarian cancer. Fortunately, she was negative.

The two of them decided they would take the most aggressive route possible. This would mean double mastectomy and chemo. As parents, they decided they would have age-appropriate discussions with the kids. They wanted to be honest and open about what was happening. They also wanted to be as positive as possible. They knew that their attitude through all this would determine how the kids would look at it.

"Mom has breast cancer. She is going to be sick. Will lose her hair. But it is **not** a death sentence. She'll be fine after all of this. Treatment will make mom sick—but she will be better in the end." They were concerned for their kids because the kids' favorite pastor at church had died of brain cancer. They shared with the kids that there are all types of cancer and that this one was not like brain cancer.

Before the surgery Heather pulled her team together at the office. Her fifteen employees (now 55) were told what was happening. Of course, tears were shed—but she was glad not to have to worry about word getting out via the grapevine.

March 5, 2013: surgery. Double mastectomy with reconstructive surgery. A lot in one day, but it was the best option.

The kids were in sports all the time. Heather and Jeffrey made the decision to keep their world as normal as possible. This meant weekends at the ballpark—whatever it took.

Three weeks after surgery, Heather was back at the office. Although the surgeries took quite a bit out of her, she managed it, chest drainage tubes and all. Her mother being able to help was, as Heather described it, a "God thing." Mom lived up North and had just retired. Instead of an insane work schedule, she had the time to come down to Texas and spend three weeks helping Heather.

At that time, too, Heather felt the hands and feet of Jesus—in her family and friends. So many people jumped to the occasion to help. One friend started a meal train and people brought food. I know this because MK was on the schedule to make and deliver dinner one night. It was a blessing for us to know that we were somehow helping.

One night at a restaurant, a woman came up to Heather and said, "God told me to come over and hug you." Heather knew things like this are not happenstance.

People that she hadn't talked to in 20 years got in touch. The entire community rallied around her.

As she started chemo, Heather learned that between the second and third chemo session she would lose her hair. She made this a fun event for the kids as she started to lose clumps of hair. She got hair shearers and had the kids shave her head. First, a mohawk with pictures. Then they shaved her bald.

Heather seldom wore wigs and scarves. Most times she went bald, even at the concession stand at the ballfield. The league uniforms all had the pink cancer awareness logo on them. Her daughter, Sara's team, held a "Hits for Heather" fundraiser one weekend to help defray costs. When the total was announced there wasn't a dry eye in the house.

The private equity partner of our company sent a picture to Heather showing them all dressed in pink on the day of her surgery. They also sent her a four-and-a-half-foot teddy bear.

Heather was amazed at the outpouring of love. For those of us who love and admire her, it was no surprise at all.

The day Heather got her diagnosis, she had one single prayer: "Lord, whatever happens with this, make something good out of it." He did and she saw Jesus in these people in so many ways.

During her surgeries, doctors discovered cancerous lymph nodes. Heather began chemo the second week of April—once every three weeks.

Chemo.

An all-day affair. The first session is the scariest, because you don't really know what to expect. God blessed her with a chemo nurse that she knew, as their daughters played ball together. Having Liz as her nurse immediately put Heather at ease. The first round went well, and she and her husband settled into a routine. Jeffrey would drop her off, go to work, come back for lunch, then pick her up at the end of the session.

When Heather wasn't sleeping, she was a social butterfly. In that six-month period, she got to know the nurses and office staff, learned about their families, and would chat with other patients. She learned that her neighbor was best friends with one of her nurses!

Her type of breast cancer was triple-positive. She would undergo six months of chemo and a year of weekly infusions. Heather felt so blessed to do her treatments near home in Waco rather than at MD Anderson in Houston—which was known as the premier cancer hospital in Texas.

Every three weeks, Heather would take a vacation day on Thursday for chemo. On Friday she'd head back to work as she felt fine. She headed to the ballpark on the weekends for her kids' games. If she got tired, she would just take a blanket and sleep on the grass. Monday and Tuesday were tough days. She was drained and would sleep 12-24 hours. More vacation days then. In all practicality Heather only took three weeks of PTO. Unbelievable!

After chemo, her dirty blonde and poker-straight hair grew back mahogany brown and curly. She always wanted curls: what a fun blessing! She joked that having chemo was like getting a perm from the inside out.

I asked Heather about her Christian upbringing to get a better idea of her faith.

Her parents divorced when she was six. She lived with her dad in Buffalo and her mom moved to Cleveland. She grew up in an Episcopalian church where she was an altar server. She remembers, however, that it never seemed sincere or fulfilling. There was a script that the priest followed each week.

Meanwhile her mom was saved and became an enthusiastic follower of Jesus. When she visited her mom, she was quite different than she'd been before. But Heather was not interested at all as her newfound religion seemed so different.

Along the way Heather eventually became a follower of Jesus but never mentioned it to anyone. Not Mom. Not Dad. No one.

Fast-forward to 1997. She was tired of the snow. Tired of being in Buffalo where the job market was scarce. She moved to the Dallas metro and found a job, where she met Jeffrey. While they were dating, she went with him to his parents' church, and she heard a Baptist minister who spoke from the heart—not from a script. She remembers telling Jeffrey she was so excited about that church.

In 1999 they got married in Lewisville, Texas, and began attending church at FBC Denton, where Heather was baptized.

They moved to Waco in 2006 and have been members of the FBC Woodway ever since. MK and I have been to that church. Amazing.

The year after surgery and chemo, a nurse was looking at her chart and mentioned to her that last year had been a bad year for her. Heather countered that it had been the most amazing year of her life. She'd felt God's blessings more in that year than any other time in her life.

Heather learned that life is about how you impact people. She often speaks with people who have gone through an experience like hers. Building trust. Sharing that life is simply about loving Jesus and loving people!

She knows that people, when in time of need, need Jesus. He isn't optional. He is someone they especially need then—and will always need for the rest of their lives.

Her concluding thoughts were about the importance of letting others in if you are faced with this or any other life-threatening, life-altering issue. So many people want to remain private. Heather said that this is the time to let others love you. Let them support you. Let them pray for you. And when you go through something hard, God can and will use you to help others.

4-year-old Thomas–High-Risk Stage IV Sarcoma

(Names have all been changed)
MK and I worked with Thomas' dad. The impact this illness had on the family – who is amazing! – is palpable today. We were always fans of Ronald McDonald House charities, and now we have a personal reason to support them.

T homas is now a junior in college. His story starts in 2007 on Halloween. As a four-year old, Thomas loved Spiderman—his favorite character. He just had to wear a Spiderman costume for trick-or-treating and get as much candy as he could. Always good to have goals as a four-year-old.

The next day Thomas told his mom and dad that his legs and stomach really hurt. Dad was sure it was from all that candy he had been carrying and how much he might have eaten. On Friday, the preschool nurses called his mom, telling her that Thomas said his hip hurt so much. That was it for Mom: off to the hospital with little Thomas.

The hospital took X-rays and said it looked as if he was bound up by his stool. Picture his dad, Pete, that Friday evening, struggling to give his four-year-old an enema.

Saturday was worse. Thomas woke up crying that his right shin was burning off. That was it. His mom, Kelly, told Pete they were taking Thomas to the children's hospital immediately. They did. The doctors knew there was something serious happening but wanted an ultrasound first.

On Sunday, less than seven days since Thomas had been Spiderman, he was diagnosed with a grapefruit-sized mass inside his stomach. Pete and Kelly were told it was malignant. Thomas was taken immediately to a room. They soon found out that it was high-risk stage IV sarcoma. A type of muscle cancer.

Initially, doctors hoped that they could surgically remove it, but they soon found that it was wrapped around the muscles in his stomach. Surgery was impossible. It had to be a combination of chemo and radiation.

Thomas's room was on the eighth floor. A wonderful room for a child. It became almost surreal for his parents as they walked in that beautiful room and saw such a beautiful sight looking out the window of the room. Next to them, their baby had no idea what he was about to go through. Neither did they.

On November 6 chemo started. This chemo would be twenty cycles of six different chemo drugs, as Pete described it, to attempt to shrink the tumor. These twenty cycles would take over 15 months to complete. During chemo would be radiation.

Thomas wouldn't be able to eat, so doctors inserted a feeding tube in his belly that stayed there for months. It would be where the young boy got all his nutrition.

After the first chemo began, Thomas showed a positive reaction. The tumor was shrinking! They were not even close to being out of the woods, but there was a relief that everything was moving in the right direction.

Kelly and Pete searched for the best hospital to provide radiation for a four-year-old with this type of stage IV cancer. Children's hospitals provided radiation, but research showed there were other types that might be best for their child.

It came down to two hospitals. They chose Memorial Sloan Kettering in New York City.

Pete was in the military. He was trained for stressful situations. He needed to be logical when in combat.

As they were planning the trip to NYC, Pete was scheduled to take off the following Monday for six months away on a deployment. The military came through with excellence! They told him to stay with his family as long as needed. He did. He will always be grateful.

Kelly and Pete had distinct roles throughout the next year. Pete was the statistician, using an Excel spreadsheet to track every chemo, every radiation, every nausea medicine, every conversation with every doctor, and every one of Thomas's reactions throughout the entire 15-month process. He had so many data points and was so well organized, he could tell Thomas how he was going to feel on day four after chemo.

Cheryl was the oncologist who performed the radiation on Thomas. It was called IMRT radiation (Intensity Modulated Radiation Therapy). Later Pete and Kelly found out that Dr. Cheryl invented the protocols for this type of radiation. Simply put, the radiation would circulate through the body until it discovered the tumor. Then, and only then, the machine would fire off the radiation directly at the tumor.

Thomas had to be medevacked from the children's hospital to Sloan Kettering in NYC. The family will be staying at Ronald McDonald House close to the hospital. RMH housed eighty-three other families sharing similar experiences. It became a petri dish of families going through the same things together.

The joys . . . the disappointments . . . the counseling . . . the grief of having a child with cancer. Volunteers for RMH provided respite for the kids as well as the parents. The kids needed a break from all the testing, treatments, and pain that the hospital provided. Some kids even got to go to Yankee games.

Parents, on the other hand, needed a break from the stress—personal and marital—that goes with having a child in the hospital and so many decisions needing to be made daily.

Kelly provided spiritual inspiration for the family. Prayers were organized with people they'd never met and had no idea how they joined the prayer warrior team. She would do all the research on alternative medicines, holistic medicines, creating positive energy, and anything else that could help heal Thomas.

The greatest stress, Pete told me, was a fear that if they came to a fork in the road, and the two of them strongly disagreed about which fork was better— then what? Something a couple never wants to go through. Thankfully, Pete and Kelly got through all those situations.

Trying to stay in shape for military duty, Pete ran each morning. Near RMH was a Catholic church. Pete had been a Catholic since in his mother's womb, he said. He eventually met Fr. Jones, a retired Navy chaplain, who began running with him. As they ran, they would stop at every Roman Catholic church they saw and light a candle and pray for his son. Soon they were looking for more churches where they could light a candle and say a prayer for Thomas.

Thomas, not in kindergarten yet, was getting great preschool tutoring from the volunteers at RMH.

In December, they started getting Christmas gift cards and other gifts that were taking up their living room. Kelly's dad told Pete, "The gift is in the giving. So many people are praying for you and sending your gift of love. Accepting them with love is the best gift you can give them in return." Advice Pete has never forgotten.

The goal was to come home for Christmas, if possible. They had been at RMH and doing radiation and chemo treatments there since February. They were blessed to make it home by Christmas and celebrate Thomas's return home.

There were still a couple of chemo sessions to finish, and fortunately, Thomas could receive treatment back at their local children's hospital.

By February all the chemo and radiation sessions were complete. At that point, the doctors declared that Thomas had "no evidence of disease." It would take five years for the doctors to proclaim that Thomas was cured. First, yearly testing had to take place. Pete refers to this as "scan-ziety" – the anxiety one goes through when the patient is going through CT scans, PET scans, or an MRI as the family waits for the results.

All of this and Thomas was still not even in kindergarten.

As they look back today, Kelly and Pete share that his healing was done by prayers, medicine, alternative and holistic medicines, and positive energy. They believe that all of this played a part for Thomas, this strapping 19-year-old today.

He played soccer and intramural basketball in high school and is as normal as any other 19-year-old young man going to college.

He was home at Christmas and had a chance to hang out with his younger brother, Christopher. Pete has since finished his 27-year Navy career and looks back with fond memories of the blessings he had.

The next time MK and I go to a Catholic church, we will light a couple of candles: one for Thomas and another one for a child whose family is staying at a RMH and needs that special prayer and angel on their shoulder—just like Pete, Kelly, Thomas, and Christopher had on theirs!

Doug's Story - A True Jesus Warrior

At the time of this event MK was Doug's VP of Operations. I was a fellow President of one of our brands. We knew Douglas and his wife, Elizabeth, very well. Just a few months before this event we went on a cruise with several of Doug and MK's franchisees. It was a very close-knit group.

The events that occurred rocked so many lives – franchisees, employees, friends at church, their three sons along with hundreds of others. Through it all Doug and Liz's faith came shining through. Eight years later many of us still wear the "God is Good All the Time" wristbands. People who see them ask where they can get one. We simply give them ours – as we have more at home.

Doug defied the odds in so many ways. When anyone else is hurting or their religion is at risk, Doug and Liz are the first ones to be Prayer Warriors for them.

It happened to us.

On June 12, 2014, MK got a call while tending to a sick mother in Washington, who was going through her own cancer battles. Doug, president of the company for which MK was vice president, had been in a horrific bicycle accident and MK needed to hurry back to run the company. Doug hit one culvert with his front tire and face planted into a second culvert while on a ride with others—one of whom was an anesthesiologist, who saved his life.

Doug was now a paraplegic: no feeling beneath his chest. His mind wasn't damaged, and his faith in God was never stronger. But he had broken all the bones in his face, his clavicle, and his sternum. MK suddenly oversaw the company—not only the staff but also all the franchise in owners North America.

One of the things I admired so much about my wife, MK, was how she handled things. Every day, after work, she would drive to the hospital and keep Doug abreast of what happened that day. Keep in mind that he was heavily sedated during this time, but she wouldn't miss a day. He was the president of the company, and she was just stepping in during the time he was off.

Some experts thought Doug would be out of work for a year, even in the hospital for six months. After time in the Waco-area hospitals, he was transferred up to Dallas. We'd visit on weekends, but she couldn't get up after work each day as it was a two-hour drive, one-way.

By September he was back on a very part-time basis. God protected his mind and his arms and hands. He could still type, communicate well, and lead.

Soon he was driving a specially outfitted van and riding a hand bike for disabled adults that he pedaled with him arms and hands.

Based on Doug's support a president's position at Five Star Painting opened right after we acquired that brand. MK was offered that position. A few years later Molly Maid—the largest of our domestic brands at Dwyer, which had become Neighborly—had an opening for a president. MK was asked to take that position. That is when we moved to Michigan: Molly Maid's headquarters were in Ann Arbor.

Doug gave so much more to people than he ever asked. No surprise when they suggested that Doug and his wife Liz Facetime us each Monday night to learn the latest development in this journey and offer a prayer. What great Christian friends!

I've always believed in prayer, and we experienced it dramatically in Doug's story. Liz never left Doug's bedside in the hospital for weeks. They would pray, sing songs (Doug would hum along), and share books. Liz read *Thrive* by Mark Hall of Casting Crowns to Doug repeatedly as he laid in the hospital after his accident. Doug also loved the song "Thrive" by Casting Crowns.

Not too long after Doug returned home from the hospital stays, Casting Crowns was playing near Waco, Texas, where we all lived. An article appeared in the Waco Tribune announcing the concert the following Friday. I reached out to the writer of the article. Crickets. He never returned my call. Never returned my email. Nothing.

When MK and I got home that night, I tried to figure out how we could get Casting Crowns to meet Doug before the show. They were so important in his healing process. I looked everywhere on social media to see how I could reach the band members.

I sent a long, impassioned e-mail to their agent and anyone else I could find associated with the band. Somehow the hand of God led me find the email addresses for band members. I sent them an email, and then we prayed about it.

Eight minutes after I sent the e-mail, Megan Garret, keyboardist, and vocalist in the band, responded they would love to meet Doug on Friday night! I looked at her reply and cried.

I told MK that God tells us to pray, we do, he answers, and we are shocked. Something is wrong with that. It was a prayer immediately answered. What we the odds that Megan was looking at her email exactly at that time?

On Friday night we met Doug and Liz at the venue and were ushered backstage. Doug and Liz shared how important Casting Crowns' music and Mark Hall's book had been during the initial stages of recovery. We also met Dave of Sidewalk Prophets and Mandisa. We still look at the pictures of all of us and marvel at God's answer to prayers.

Yes, we are huge fans of Christian music now. We've seen many of the artists. And, yes, we are even bigger fans of prayer.

Stephen-Leukemia with a Bone Marrow Transplant

I forget how Stephen and I got introduced. It wasn't until the end of our discussion that I found out that he works for a supplier our company worked very closely with. My previous VP and Stephen are great friends. Stephen remembers meeting Mary Kay at our annual convention years ago.

Small world. And, as you are about to learn, the world gets even smaller. This is a must-read for anyone who ever gets a bad diagnosis in their life. You will learn how important a positive attitude is, along with a belief that things will eventually be good regardless of how long it takes.

Amazing and inspirational. Whatever situation you think you can't get through read Stephen's story and think again.

Stud athlete. The first words that come to mind when I think about Stephen in his college days. A pitcher for Rice University in Houston. Drafted by Major League Baseball his junior year. Decides to come back and finish his degree at Rice. Selected in the MLB draft his senior year by the Detroit Tigers.

He entered the Detroit farm system in 1999 as a 6'4" relief pitcher. Had the aggressive and competitive attitude of "put me in the game with the bases loaded, nobody out, we are only up by one run, and I'll get out of this" every time he went out to the mound to pitch. He thrives on pressure situations. Hurt his arm after three seasons, had Tommy John surgery, and that was the end of his professional sports career. As a college and pro athlete, he learned to know his body through minor injuries that always healed, given enough time. The injury he would have post-baseball was one he was not prepared for.

Jump to the early fall of 2012. He was thirty-five and still in great shape. Swam and lifted weights several times per week at a local gym. While lap swimming one day it felt like someone had shot him in the hip. There was a white-hot, searing intense pain. Stephen saw his local sports medicine doctor for a general work-up. The doctor says it's just a sports injury and recommends Advil and general rest to allow it to heal. But a week later, he felt as if it was getting worse. Stephen found it difficult to lift his leg to enter his vehicle to drive. In the back of his mind, Stephen knew something was wrong.

Stephen returned to the sports medicine doctor and said, "I know something is not right here. I've been an athlete my entire life and this feels like a different type of pain and injury to me." The doctor ordered X-rays and an MRI. All came back clean.

On Stephen's third trip to the doctor, the doctor ordered a CT scan. The scan came back abnormal, but the orthopedic doctor wasn't sure what the problem was. He referred Stephen to another local doctor—this time, an oncologist. It was approaching Thanksgiving 2012, three months after the initial symptoms.

The oncologist ordered blood tests, and all came back clean. However, the CT scan showed diffused (broad) imaging in Stephen's bones, so the oncologist performed a bone marrow biopsy in the office under local anesthesia. This is an excruciatingly painful test where a sharp metal rod is jammed into the lower lumbar/hip area to remove bone marrow (the spongy material inside one's bones that creates your blood and houses your immune system). The results shocked the oncologist: Stephen was diagnosed with Acute Lymphoblastic Leukemia (ALL). It's an aggressive form of blood cancer that is most prevalent in adolescents and elderly patients. It's a highly unusual blood cancer for someone his age.

The doctor suggested immediate admission into the hospital, saying that, had this gone undiagnosed much longer, Stephen would have passed away within months. If ever there were an example of why it is critical for patients to know their body, and to advocate for themselves without compromise, it's Stephen. A blood test only a few days after the bone marrow biopsy finally showed leukemia cells in Stephen's blood stream. Much like baseball is a game of inches, Stephen's health journey was now coming down to a matter of days. He was quickly admitted into City of Hope, a world-renowned cancer hospital in Los Angeles, for immediate treatment.

At this time Stephen and his wife were trying to start a family. She, too, was a college athlete who became a hospital pharmacist. This was both a blessing and a bit of a curse in that she understood the diagnosis very well. She understood all the medications and chemo Stephen would have to take and knew the prognosis as well. It was grim, but not terminal.

Stephen asked his hematologist at City of Hope, "Can a human being survive this?"

She said, "Yes, it's possible, but it will be a long and very difficult road."

Stephen said, "If one person has ever survived this, I will survive this too; let's get started."

Treatment immediately began, with a 30-day induction cycle to get Stephen into remission via intense chemo treatments.

The chemo to treat ALL is intense and concentrated and consists of multiple chemotherapies fed into the bloodstream. There was one particularly nasty chemo Stephen remembers called Daunorubicin—a red chemo that can cause third-degree burns if it touches skin. They administered it through a central line in Stephen's artery, directly into his blood stream, while the nurses wore hazmat suits. The chemo began killing every cancer cell in his body, as well as his healthy cells. Stephen's blood count dropped, his hair fell out, and his energy levels went to zero.

Most people don't realize that chemo isn't mass-produced. It is made in the pharmacy specifically for that person's issues, their body weight, type of cancers, and so forth. Stephen learned this when his wife told him she had mastered this in pharmacy school, even getting an award for it.

Doctors inserted a venous catheter into Stephen that was used not only for the chemo to be inserted in his body, but also to withdraw blood. This remained in his body for two years.

After a month in the hospital, Stephen was released to go home for Christmas. He was so weak that he had to crawl on his hands and knees to get up the stairs into the bedroom. During his brief recovery, Stephen says he cried himself to sleep most nights; not from sadness or feeling sorry for himself, but due to the frustration. Cancer had brought his entire life to a complete halt. The people he loved the most were all grieving his illness, some unsure what to say, some not saying anything, and others simply weeping when talking to him or being around him.

A doctor at City of Hope is famous for saying, "Cancer is a thief. It steals your time, it steals your health, and it steals your energy. But it can never steal your hope." Stephen was determined to see this through and to get to the other side, but the worst was yet to come.

In early 2013, Stephen returned to the hospital for a longer, second round of chemo. As this began, the doctor said that to survive long-term, Stephen would need a bone marrow transplant to replace Stephen's diseased bone marrow with healthy bone marrow from an unrelated but genetically matched donor. The global search for Stephen's donor began, organized through City of Hope and Be the Match (bethematch.org).

Human leukocyte antigen (HLA) typing is used to match patients and donors for bone marrow or cord blood transplants. HLA are proteins or markers, found on most cells in your body. Your immune system uses these markers to recognize which cells belong in your body and which do not.

Stephen describes the wait as excruciating. He knew he could not survive on chemo and blood transfusions forever. He needed an HLA-matched donor fast.

There are 10 HLAs that can be matched. Doctors located a perfect match for Stephen, a 10-out-of-10 match. Only one problem: he was in Germany. The coordination to obtain the donor's stem cells at the same time Stephen was prepared to receive them was, as Stephen described it, like hitting a bullseye on a stationary target while shooting out of a car traveling at one hundred miles per hour. The timing was everything.

To prepare for the bone marrow transplant, Stephen had to be brought as close to death as possible; his entire immune system had to be destroyed. Treatment was a combination of high-dose chemo and full-body radiation. Many patients pass away from the treatment, not the cancer itself, at this point because it is so aggressive. For a month Stephen survived on blood transfusions, platelet transfusions, whole red blood cells, and various other blood products while the alignment of his donor's cell donation and Stephen's journey to absolute zero came together.

The radiation was so intense that it had to be spread over multiple treatments per day over several days. Stephen asked, "Can you just give it to me all at once?" and the radiation oncologist said quite plainly, "Sir, that would kill you." So, over a week's period, Stephen received radiation over his entire body (while hanging from a hazmat suit.) Many patients pass out during these treatments, as well as intense intravenous chemotherapy. He was vomiting often. They put him on IV fluids and nutrition because he could not hold food down.

The cells arrived from Germany on April 16th, but not in the morning as they anticipated. The long day's wait finally concluded after 10 p.m., when a tiny bag of yellow stem cells was delivered to Stephen's hospital room and given to him via an IV line. Stephen describes the experience as one of the most anticlimactic events of his life! Laughing while retelling the story, Stephen recalls, "For some reason, all the anticipation and buildup to this moment had me imagining myself in a room with fireworks going off, flashing lights, perhaps a few dancers tumbling around the room— you know, a Super Bowl type of event scene. Of course, that's not at all what happened. The nurses walked into the room, showed me the bag of cells, and my doctor confidently said, 'Stephen, this is what's going to save you.' I was teetering between being overjoyed and being so exhausted that I couldn't muster up the energy to even cry. It was surreal. After about 20 minutes, the transfusion was complete."

Then, it was the "hurry up and wait" part of the recovery. The new stem cells had to graft into Stephen's bones where his old bone marrow used to be. Every couple of hours Stephen's blood was drawn to check for progress, and for signs of the countless ways this procedure could go wrong. It was a week before the cells grafted and Stephen's blood counts began to increase. His new bone marrow was being created, and his body had begun to create its own blood. Only now Stephen had his donor's bone marrow, which meant his body was now creating his donor's blood.

For bone marrow transplant patients, the first one hundred days of post-transplant are critical. There are more complications than Stephen could recount but suffice it to say that this time period is one of intense oversight by doctors and nurses. Stephen was in his hospital room for 43 days while his marrow was grafted. For the next one hundred days he would be in housing on the campus of City of Hope because of all the blood tests that were needed and the many complications that could occur. It was imperative he was close in case there were any issues.

When I asked Stephen where he got his inspiration for handling this all with grace, he told of a mentor he had in high school. His junior year, his English teacher was also the headmaster of his all-boys school in Nashville. Midyear this teacher was diagnosed with terminal pancreatic cancer.

He taught for the remainder of the year. Never complained. No one would have guessed he was dying. The teacher was a Rhodes Scholar. Brilliant. Stephen learned so much from him about handling adversity that year before he passed away at the too-young age of fifty.

Interacting with his teacher during this time taught Stephen about dealing with challenges with grace, humility, and even humor. Stephen took these learnings into his own cancer experience and made it a point to have his nurses and his doctor laughing much more often than they were being serious. Stephen says his sense of humor is what kept him from getting too down, while his competitiveness kept him striving for the next milestone in his recovery.

"Attitude is everything in a situation like that," he said, "because you're surrounded by other patients who may not have the same chances you do, or have the same mental outlook you do, and it's all too easy to start feeling sorry for yourself. I refused to do that except in the most extreme and fleeting moments. I knew I had to survive because my family and my wife expected it. I couldn't let them down."

The transition happening within Stephen's body was miraculous. His body was creating his donor's blood now, which meant his blood type changed from O-negative to A-positive. Our allergies are stored in our bone marrow and immune system, which meant Stephen's allergies changed; his donor was not allergic to cats, meaning Stephen managed to lose his explosive cat allergy thanks to his new bone marrow. A heck of a way to lose an allergy, but Stephen laughed and said he'd take the benefits from this where he could get them.

When Stephen was able to go home, his body ached. A simple cold felt like a truck hit him. His body was adjusting to his new insides. There is always a chance the donor's blood might not adapt to the recipient' organs. Stephen didn't have any of these issues except for a slight issue in his stomach. Given the circumstances, this was a miracle.

Stephen's progress was monitored through countless blood tests; daily for months, then every other day, then less frequently, until he finally was healthy enough to get monthly checkups for several years. During this initial recovery, Stephen received a dozen bone marrow biopsies as well to check his DNA and genetics to ensure he remained in remission.

It took over two years to go back to work and longer until he could start working out again. Just walking without getting out of breath was workout enough at first.

After ten years now, he must only go to the doctor every six to nine months. He describes this as a check-up frequency he never would have imagined, especially in the early parts of his recovery when they were checking him hourly. "To say I am blessed and fortunate is an understatement; what I went through is often not survived, and those of us who do survive are often dealing with lifelong side effects and increases in risks for treatment-caused cancers and organ failures that in and of themselves are enormous challenges. I know my crazy competitiveness helped me get through this. A doctor told me 'The body follows the mind,' and to a huge extent, I agree. I am living proof of that."

City of Hope celebrates its survivors with an annual bone marrow survivors' reunion, as well as an annual celebrity softball fundraiser event in Nashville. Stephen was invited to Nashville to attend the event in 2015. The timing coincided with the Country Music Festival, and stars like Vince Gill were playing in the game. Being from Nashville, Stephen was honored at a chance to go home.

Stephen was brought onto the field with his wife—now pregnant!—to watch a video on the video scoreboard that City of Hope had recorded with him months before. At the conclusion of the video, Stephen and his wife Erin turned around, and there stood Jonas, Stephen's bone marrow donor. City of Hope had flown Jonas in from Germany to meet Stephen in person, on the field, in front of thousands of people in the stands at the game. Stephen and Jonas hugged, and the crowd erupted. Tears flowed. Stephen recalls, "How on earth do you find adequate words to say 'thank you' to someone who helped save your life—via a selfless donation to a person he did not know at the time? I hugged Jonas about as tight as I've ever hugged someone, looked him in the eye, and just said 'Thank you Jonas. I'm here right now because of you.' We have become good friends since that day. I still tear up thinking about that moment."

At another City of Hope fundraiser at a preseason Dodgers game, Stephen told his story from home plate with over 20,000 in attendance. He played catch with the president of City of Hope on the field in front of the fans.

Stephen describes himself as a very spiritual person. Growing up in the South, he was surrounded by religion at every turn, but he knows there is an indescribable spiritual component to his survival as well.

Stephen said, "I believe in God, I know there is more to our existence than we understand, because as I went through this cancer ordeal, I could feel it when people were praying for me. I don't know how to describe it, other than feeling a warmth, a deep love and care in my heart and soul that I hadn't felt so intensely before all of this. I have no doubt that the energy we put out into the world matters; it affects not only ourselves but more importantly it affects others. I can never thank my friends, and my friends' friends, and my family, for praying for me, for sending positive energy out into the world for me, and for just loving me the way they did during this experience. I couldn't have made it without them."

Of course, he said, something like this can test one's faith. But it never took him away.

It is important to Stephen to share these concluding thoughts:

Cancer is not a death sentence. The procedure that saved his life wasn't invented until the year he was born: 1976. Medicine continues to advance, and fundraisers for cancer research matter. Please donate when you can.

If you're healthy, consider becoming a donor.

Become a blood donor: blood is always needed locally. Donate when you can.

- Become a potential life-saving donor by signing up with Be the Match (Marrow.org)
- Donate your time at hospitals: you never know when just a smile can help a cancer patient get through the day.

Attitude matters. The mental toll a cancer diagnosis takes is devastating, but it does not have to destroy your hope. It's OK to have bad days. But never, ever, *ever* give up. Never.

Rather than asking a patient "is there anything I can do to help?" ask instead, "I am going to do something to help you while you're going through this. What would you like me to do?" And if the patient can't think of an answer, choose something to do for them on your own. They will always remember even the smallest thing you do to help them.

If you're unsure what to say to a friend or family member who has been diagnosed with cancer, please do not choose to say nothing at all. Even a few simple words like, "I don't know what to say, but I do want you to know I love you/I care about you" will make a world of difference to the recipient. As a patient going through this, Stephen was shocked to discover years later that there were people who just chose to not reach out at all because they didn't know what to say. Say something, anything. Cancer patients need as much support as they can get.

Sharon & Breast Cancer–Single Mastectomy

1984. Joan and I were going through a divorce. I moved in with my best friend to give Joan space in the hopes we could save the marriage. My best friend was dating an amazing young woman several years younger than us. She was someone that I could relate to on a faith basis, but when it came to faith, the two of them weren't on the same page. He and I attended her graduation as she earned her AA from Malone College, a private Christian university in Canton, Ohio.

After my divorce, I learned that the two of them had broken up. She was the first person I took to dinner. No romantic sparks, but we became great friends. Ours would be a special lifelong friendship.

She went on to meet and marry the right person for her and they have been married for over 30 years. A few years ago, I learned she had breast cancer. As I drafted this book, I knew I needed to talk with her. Sharon's story gives someone who is diagnosed an idea of what they might go through. The great news is that Sharon is alive, cancer-free, and living a wonderful life!

After a routine mammogram in April 2018, Sharon received a letter stating that everything looked fine and that they would see her in a year. At the time of the mammogram, Sharon had been experiencing nipple discharge from her right breast.

She researched it, and everything she read said it was nothing for which to be concerned. The discharge was clear or milky in color. The mammogram technician had told her that she should consult her doctor if she noticed a change in the discharge. And that is what happened: the discharge turned red, which meant blood. That started the events of the next two months, which included numerous doctor visits, tests, and biopsies.

Breast cancer. The phrase is scary to someone who never thought that cancer would be a problem. The phrase was scary to Sharon. Being a very private person, she chose to share the news with only her husband, her children, a best friend in Texas, and her boss. It was so personal to her that she never talked to anyone about it until after her surgery. But that didn't mean that it wasn't on her mind constantly.

Initially her surgeon recommended a lumpectomy. But, after further tests, the surgeon determined that a mastectomy would be the better plan since the cancer cells were widespread throughout the breast. Sharon also met with a plastic surgeon to discuss options for reconstruction. Instead of choosing to have an implant, which she had heard horror stories about, she opted to have a TRAM flap. TRAM stands for transverse rectus abdominis muscle, tissue used to replace breast tissue.

The more she learned about what was about to happen, she remembered Philippians 4:6-7:

> Do not be anxious about anything, but in every situation, by prayer and petition, with thanksgiving, present your requests to God. And the peace of God, which transcends all understanding, will guard your hearts and your minds in Christ Jesus.

A full recovery would require two major surgeries. And Sharon was about to learn that the TRAM flap surgery was much more difficult than the mastectomy itself.

As she looked in the mirror, 2 Corinthians 12:9 popped into her head:

"My grace is sufficient for you, for my power is made perfect in weakness." Therefore, I will boast all the more gladly about my weaknesses, so that Christ's power may rest on me.

The surgery was in September 2018. The surgeon did the mastectomy and then the plastic surgeon immediately followed with the TRAM flap and reconstruction. She was recovering from two major surgeries: she had five drain tubes and was in the hospital for a week. She recalls sitting in a chair in her hospital room in tears and crying out to God, telling Him she couldn't do this recovery alone. He gave her the Scripture in 2 Corinthians 12:9: *"My grace is sufficient for you, for my power is made perfect in weakness."* She knew God truly was with her every step of the way.

Some people get mad at God when they hear the news of a serious health challenge. Not Sharon. She didn't ask, why me? Instead, she thought, why *not* me? She knows that we live in a sinful world and terrible things happen.

She also knows that this isn't as good as it gets. This world is not our home. Someday we will be in heaven where there will be no more sickness or death. But until then we live with the effects of a fallen world.

She continually prayed, "God, help me learn what you want me to learn with all of this—and if I can help someone with what I'm going through, then help me do this."

Amazing faith.

Her children's reaction was wonderful. But it was difficult for them at first. The words "cancer" and "mom" don't go together.

Sharon's daughter, Alyssa, lived down the street, within walking distance of Sharon's house. Alyssa came over every day with her one-year-old son and cleaned her mom's wound and applied fresh bandages. She emptied and measured her drain tubes and took Mom to her doctor's appointments. Alyssa set up a meal train for two weeks. Sharon said, "I was overwhelmed at the response and felt incredibly blessed by people who brought meals." Sharon explains that she couldn't have done it without her wonderful daughter who was such a blessing during that time!

An in-home nurse came twice a week, and Sharon received physical therapy at home every two weeks.

During the healing process Sharon noticed the wound wasn't healing. She was suffering skin necrosis, meaning the skin had died. Next up was a skin graft from the skin on her thigh.

Before surgery they tell you not to eat or drink after midnight the day before. Her surgery for the skin graft wasn't until later in the day and by that time Sharon was dehydrated. The nurse tried three times to get the IV in and couldn't, so she called the anesthesiologist. He tried four times and ended up using an ultrasound machine to find a vein.

She was lying there with tears streaming down her face. She vividly remembers the awful pain! The anesthesiologist told her that if she ever needed to have another surgery to make sure she had fluids up to three or four hours before the procedure!

This all meant a longer healing time. A longer time away from work. 12 weeks in total.

In February 2019 Sharon went in for a breast reduction on the left side so both breasts would match. That was a much easier recovery process.

After surgeries, Sharon was referred to an oncologist at a well-known cancer center. The first time Sharon saw her, this doctor walked into the room with a laptop. She did not know anything about her case. She read her computer and asked a question here and there. She was very impersonal with terrible bedside manners. She said she wanted Sharon to go on medicine for five to ten years. She named two different medicines and proceeded to list all the negative side effects, which could also include death! Then she asked which one Sharon wanted to take! There was no compassion, no empathy.

This is a lesson I learned from Sharon. If you ever feel that you are seeing the wrong doctor, **you are**! Find someone you trust. Someone you can trust to put your life in their hands . . . and heart!

Sharon left there feeling frightened and confused. She had one more visit and then changed oncologists. She had heard wonderful things about a different oncologist and made an appointment with him. At their first meeting, he walked into the room without a laptop and just told her that he was familiar with her case. He said that in her situation he believed that the risks of the medicine outweighed the benefits, so he recommended that she not take anything. She followed his advice!

Sharon went for a mammogram every six months to keep an eye on things. In the summer of 2022, she went in for a routine mammogram and they saw an area of concern on the left breast. They did a needle biopsy and then scheduled Sharon for a surgical biopsy. The surgeon prepared her, explaining that she would have to go on medicine and go back to the oncologist. The doctor was expecting to find cancer and she wanted to prepare Sharon.

On the day of the surgical biopsy, Sharon left the house about 5 a.m. She was following her husband because they were dropping his car off at the shop before continuing to the hospital. It was still dark outside. Suddenly Sharon felt tingling in her left breast, right where they were going to do the biopsy. She had never felt anything quite like that before. Sharon said aloud, "Jesus, are you healing me?!"

The result of the biopsy: they found nothing! To this day Sharon believes that Jesus healed her that morning on the way to the hospital! So, no medicine and no visits to the oncologist!

I asked Sharon for advice for others diagnosed with breast cancer.

Take one day at a time. She received her diagnosis in July and didn't have surgery until September.

- You'll think about this every day. At work. At home. When you wake up. When you go to sleep. This is normal.
- Don't make it worse than it is by imagining the worst.
- God will give you the grace when you need it.
- If you have an oncologist, you don't like or you don't trust, change oncologists.

If you have a friend or relative who is dealing with a cancer diagnosis, please tell them you are praying for them or thinking about them. The journey is lonely.

No one else knows what you are going through, but knowing they are there praying for you helps. When Sharon's sister contracted breast cancer, she told Sharon, "I didn't understand. If I would have, I would have been there much more for you."

No one can ever convince Sharon that there aren't miracles—she had one.

Case #6:

Kirklyn-Colon Cancer

Kirklyn Dixon is a franchisee for a well-known company. His story is an unusual one. One about colon cancer. One about survival. One about prayer.

Sunday night was always date night for Kirklyn and his wife, Denise. They loved looking forward to Sunday dinner out and deciding where they would go.

On October 29, 2017, Kirklyn noticed that Outback Steakhouse had a special. He loved red meat and saw that on this Sunday night they had a special hamburger dinner. Special seasonings. Looked delicious.

The advertisements were correct. It was delicious. But right after dinner, Kirklyn felt ill. It wasn't food poisoning; the meat had been perfectly cooked. It must have been something else. He told Denise he was going to run to the bathroom and be right back.

The second he seated himself on the toilet, blood ran out. Spattered everywhere. Pure blood—not anything else. The bathroom was full of blood.

Kirklyn is a man's man. No doctors. No hospitals. But he called Denise on his phone from the bathroom and told her to hurry and pay the check. They were going directly to the hospital—just a couple of miles away.

As they entered the hospital the staff did all the things an ER staff does. Have a seat, we will be right with you. They would then do all the paperwork and, finally, the patient would head back to ER. Kirklyn told the staff he needed to see a doctor—NOW!

He then headed straight to the ER's restroom and the same thing happened. Pure blood. Sprayed throughout the restroom. Filling the stool. The staff finally understood that he needed to get into an exam room, posthaste.

He and Denise went back to a triage room that, fortunately, had a bathroom shared with the next room. Again, the same thing happened. Blood everywhere in the bathroom.

Denise had called one of Kirklyn's best friends. When Kirklyn came back into the room, his friend was there with Denise. He lay down, told his wife the room was getting dark, and passed out. Doctors had to revive him.

He was admitted immediately into ICU. The doctor said he would be re-evaluated Monday and that he would have a colonoscopy.

When the doctor came in, he and Kirklyn discovered they shared a common love. Both were graduates of Georgia Tech. They bonded immediately, and Kirklyn trusted the doctor.

Tuesday's colonoscopy wasn't good. The doctor found polyps and a growth. He explained that he had seen this before. In most cases it means cancer. The surgery was scheduled for the next day.

After surgery, the doctor came in and confirmed the worst. He told Kirklyn and Denise, "It's cancer." Kirklyn remembers that he and Denise had a calmness about them that most doctors don't see when they break this news. Simple for them: it was their faith in God. Both were active in their church. God was with them.

The doctor was concerned because of the size of the tumor. He explained that the bleeding Kirklyn experienced had saved his life because it bled so profusely. The cancer didn't get into his bloodstream or any other organs.

After more tests they labeled his cancer stage IIIA. In plain language this means the cancer hasn't gotten out of the organ and into the bloodstream.

Surgeons removed the entire tumor and part of the tissue on the sides of the tumor. Yes, the surrounding lymph nodes contained cancer cells. Chemo was ordered to make sure everything left was taken care of.

Chemo couldn't be started until there had been four weeks of "clean time," just to make sure none of the incisions got infected.

The largest of the four did. This meant that chemo would have to be postponed and the doctor would have to go back in to clean up the infection. Denise cleaned the wound daily as it healed.

Chemo started January 10, 2018.

Kirklyn received chemo every other Wednesday. He had a pump that continued to slowly release chemo for two more days. He could take off the bag of chemicals late Friday afternoons.

His amazing work ethic compelled him to keep up at work through the treatments. He was worn out but still worked every Thursday and Friday. Coworkers supported him and understood if he just had to put his head down for a moment or two.

Still, Kirklyn drove himself to work.

The doctor warned Kirklyn that nothing would taste good. He wouldn't be able to use silverware because it would create a bitter metallic aftertaste. He couldn't drink anything cold.

On Wednesday afternoon, though, right after chemo every two weeks, he was ready to eat. His taste buds were back for a day, and he was ready for a feast—albeit with plastic tableware.

Until the following Tuesday, Kirklyn wouldn't be able to taste anything. Nothing would taste good. For survival he could eat chicken noodle soup and broth—but it had to be as hot as possible.

Of course, he evaluated all of this and found out the doctor was right! No more silverware—only plastic! Over the chemo period he dropped forty pounds.

Saturdays after chemo were horrid. Most times he couldn't even hold his head up. After the seventh chemo session, he was fully drained. The lowest point of his life. He was tired of the chemo. He was tired of the every-other-Wednesday sessions.

At that low point, Kirklyn describes what Denise did as the most humane thing that had ever been done for him. She told him to get in the car, put the window down, and enjoy the wind and the sunshine. They drove with no destination in mind. Denise had no idea where they were going—she just wanted to be with him and share the sunshine.

She didn't talk. Just drove. Denise remembered something Kirklyn shared at one time called "the Spirit of Presence." It was something he'd learned years before. The Spirit of Presence was about how people need the presence of someone around them. They don't need advice, they don't need questions, they simply need someone to be with them. This is what she did that day. Kirklyn felt he was more loved than ever before.

He wasn't enjoying his job anymore in June of 2018 and was searching. He had always wanted to work for himself and had looked at several franchise opportunities. On June 23, 2018, while getting to ring the bell at the hospital for completing his chemo sessions, a franchise opportunity popped up on his phone. It looked remarkably interesting.

He visited the franchise, lined up SBA financing, and, in July of 2019, he bought the territory and started his new life. He was finally working for himself!

Kirklyn never had a fear of dying. He and Denise never talked about the what ifs. They never thought anything bad. Naturally during chemo, he would get discouraged, but he knew this, too, would pass.

Faith. The only way he can describe their feelings.

Initially he needed an annual colonoscopy. As of June of 2022, he needs one only every three years. He feels great.

Oh, one thing: he still eats with plastic. He only uses solo cups and plastic silverware. When he goes to fine dining, he still asks for plastic.

It will be five years soon. He is a cancer thriver, not just a cancer survivor. Faith continues to get Kirklyn and Denise through any challenges they face. They already beat the biggest one.

My last conversation was a very emotional one for Kirklyn as they reviewed their own story and remembered those times that were so difficult. They knew then, as every day, God's love, and the miracle they received in their own lives.

Case #7:

Lisa-Stage IV Hodgkin's Lymphoma

MK and I met Lisa through her husband, Steve. He was president of one of our sister brands. We met at all the Christmas parties, conventions, and get-togethers. We have even been to a party in their home.

We knew there was something special about her. We just did not know what yet.

This chapter of the book will be different. It is about someone who is currently going through cancer treatments . As I interviewed Lisa, she and Steve were on their way to MD Anderson in Houston. U.S. News and World Report has identified them as one of the best hospitals for cancer care in the U.S.

It is over three hours from their home to Houston, which is becoming their second home (not by choice). Her cancer is rare: she is one of only three in the world currently living with her condition.

I t all started on February 11, 2022. Lisa went to urgent care as she was throwing up and had constant diarrhea. Neither would stop. Urgent care sent her to the hospital thinking it was her gallbladder causing the issues. After a week, they ran through all kinds of tests. Doctors *thought* it was a bad reaction to an antibiotic. She was sent to a liver specialist because the doctors at the hospital thought that the antibiotic had caused some liver damage.

More tests with the hepatologist. He wasn't sure what she had, but he could see that there was damage to the liver based on blood tests. It was determined that her bilirubin was high. Bilirubin passes through the liver

35

and is eventually excreted out of the body. Higher than usual levels of bilirubin may indicate liver or bile duct problems. She remembers that the levels should be between 0.1 and 1.0. Hers exceeded twenty-five. Yes, an area of real concern.

He recommended that she see an oncologist. Oncologist determined that she did not have cancer, but chemotherapy was out of the question based on her damaged liver. She was sent home again to wait and see. The herpetologist kept an eye on her liver through weekly blood tests which continued to show damage to the liver. Overall, the liver was functioning, but showed signs of damage.

Lisa was sent to a hospital in the Dallas/Fort Worth area. She was there for several days, but the medical team couldn't figure out what was happening to her body.

By this time Lisa was exhausted. Her skin was yellow. Her eyes were yellow—to the point of kids noticing it in the school where she worked. "How come your eyes are so yellow, Ms. Lisa?" She lost thirty pounds, without trying, in five weeks.

Her bilirubin jumped up to 25.7. Lisa started itching. Constantly. All over her body. It reminded Steve of a gorilla in a zoo. Lisa got medicines, more medicines, creams, and anything else that might help with this itching.

Her liver specialist said, "Don't leave the hospital in Fort Worth until they know what is wrong with you." She met with the gastroenterologist, oncologist, and every other kind of "-ist" to see if they could figure out what her problem really was.

Doctors did a bone marrow biopsy. Inconclusive. Lymph nodes were inconclusive. She finally noticed a lymph node in her neck that was really swollen. She asked them to evaluate that specific lymph node and do one more bone marrow biopsy.

Viola. After 25 nights in the hospital, Lisa had an answer: the doctors concluded it was stage IV Hodgkin's lymphoma—overly aggressive.

It was then, but only then, that Lisa realized they were really telling her she had cancer. Lisa, wife, and mother of three, really had the big C word!

On top of that, her liver was out of whack. But they couldn't do a liver transplant because of the cancer! She then learned that she had paraneo-plastic syndrome, a rare disorder that occurs when the immune system has a reaction to a cancerous tumor. In lay terms: cancer is going out from the lymph nodes to attack other organs.

Along with all of this, she also had vanishing bile duct syndrome—an uncommon, acquired, but potentially serious form of chronic cholestatic liver disease. This means that her bile ducts were disappearing. One does not have life without bile ducts.

Whew.

What all of this really comes down to is that Lisa was one of a few people in the world who had all these issues. Doctors wanted to control the cancer before anything else happened.

Suddenly, she went from two pills a day to eleven. Doctors decided to do "baby chemo" treatments to see how she managed this. The doctors' thought immunotherapy was the right way to go. One of the immunotherapies rec-ommended was **not** covered under insurance.

Only one hospital in Texas is well-known as THE place to go to if you have cancer – MD Anderson in Houston. They are world-renowned.

Doctors at MD Anderson redid all the tests to make sure that the diag-noses were correct. Thankfully, once she was admitted, the medicines that were turned down by the insurance companies were now covered.

By this time, Lisa—5'6"—was down to 125 pounds. Huge weight loss is typical for lymphoma. The doctors in Houston wanted to build back her weight to see how she could tolerate the chemo treatments she was about to get.

Treatment started slowly to see how Lisa's body managed it. First, they tried a half dose. Lots of blood tests followed. All went well.

The challenge was that each portion of the ABVD affected a different part of the body.

By this time, Lisa realized that she needed to retire. Steve was thinking the same thing. The family goal was for Lisa to survive and live an amazing life—without cancer treatments. This would take time—and total commitment from them both.

Full-strength chemo was next. There were side effects. Mouth sores that extended down the throat. Total exhaustion. Every chemo dose put her back in the hospital for a couple of days.

Today, she is preparing for her next round of chemo. She'll go home after chemo as she is an outpatient. Yes, she has nausea and exhaustion—but overall, no more than expected. It is so much easier for the family, being an outpatient. She only had to go into the hospital for the first three doses. Twice a week to Houston for chemo as well as doctor appointments.

The itching is gone. Her liver numbers, which were once 25.3, are now 3.3. Not where they want them to be but really heading in the right direction.

Because her combination of illnesses is so rare, her doctors at MD Anderson consult with doctors throughout the world. How comforting this is for Lisa and Steve that they are getting the best available care in the world.

One doctor said, without thought, that Lisa would be a case study—*if* she survives. Lisa quickly corrected him: I **will** survive. You mean *as* I survive.

Awaiting her is an autologous stem cell transplant. This means harvesting Lisa's own bone marrow and transplanting it into her own body. She will have little, if any, risk of rejection because of this decision.

Lisa's stem cell treatment will require her to live in a sterile room. Steve can join her—but no one else. People can visit, but they will be staring through a window. Or they can FaceTime her.

A year after the stem cell transplant, she will start to feel normal. But a couple of months after the transplant she will start to feel better.

When this happens, and she knows it will, she will be cured of cancer.

I learned from Lisa that the liver is an amazing organ. It self-repairs and is self-healing. This means she will be back to how she was pre-2021. That is when we last saw her—a vivacious, excited person!

The biggest surprise Lisa encountered was when letting family know about her condition. Her nephews and nieces both lost a mom to breast cancer and a father, who smoked, to lung cancer. They lost both parents to the Big C. To them, cancer meant only one thing: death. To Lisa, Steve, and their kids (25-year-old son and 23-year-old twin daughters), it was simply a setback. Yes, a challenge. But that's it.

This is something that I should have put first in this story, not last. It had been the guiding force in Lisa's life.

Throughout our conversation she kept mentioning her relationship with God.

Lisa has attended church since she was a kid. She was attending Baylor University when one of her friends told her about a church she had gone to the week before that she thought Lisa would enjoy.

At that church, this 19-year-old cool college kid walked down the aisle to accept Jesus. Tough choice for a college kid to make in front of friends. Yet, she did it.

Lisa told me of one night after her diagnosis ago lying in a hospital bed. No one in the room. Suddenly, she felt a presence in her room. Extremely hard to describe it. But very real. She felt a hand on her thigh. A comforting hand.

In the next couple of days, the word *child* kept coming to her. She felt the hand and the message were telling her that she was a child of Jesus, and He would take care of her like a father takes care of his children. It might not be on this earth. Even if not, surely it would be so when she meets Him in Heaven. What a wonderful picture for Lisa.

What a wonderful picture for anyone going through what Lisa has been going through.

Case #8:

Nard-ALS & a Love Story

*Nard. Burnie. Bunz. Bill. All the same person. My broth-
er-in-law . . . MK's older brother—a year and nine days older.
Following the two of them were four more girls. Navy brats—
having to move every two years as dad's orders changed. He
was the commander of a secret spy ship.*
*Burnie, MK, and the kids, the two of them called themselves.
When I first met dad as MK and I started to date, he told me
about each of the girls. Then told me a story about his only son
– about an article that appeared in Dear Abby. Nard was a
free spirit. Dad retired in Las Vegas where he was the Junior
ROTC instructor. Each of the kids at one point lived in Vegas.
That is where Burnie met Pat. She was a lifesaver and his lifelong mate of 46 years. When people asked him how Pat was,
he simply answered, "Perfect."*

We knew the news wasn't good when Nard was diagnosed with ALS.
But from that moment, he and Pat chose to focus on living life to
the fullest. Frustrations along the way for Pat—many! But none with any
medical staff, none with Nard. Just a bunch of paperwork.

Before that time all I knew about ALS was the Ice Bucket Challenge
from the summer of 2014 and the Lou Gehrig speech, "I consider myself
the luckiest man, etc." Gehrig gave that speech on June 19, 1939 after it was
confirmed he had amyotrophic lateral sclerosis after just six days of extensive testing at the clinic. Gehrig died June 2, 1941 – just two years later

after prognosis. The $100 we contributed to the Ice Bucket challenge was a pittance.

I learned that pneumonia is typical in ALS patients, as the disease causes progressive degeneration of the voluntary muscles movements that include breathing. His doctor explained it feels like you are drowning – you can't catch your breath. One source describes ALS:

> *Many patients are unable to walk or use crutches in the late stages of ALS and require a wheelchair and assistance moving around. This is due to paralysis of the limbs caused by the disease attacking the muscles. Many also experience an inability to talk, eat or drink and require a feeding tube. (He had been on one for over a year.) There is no cure for ALS, and the disease is eventually fatal.*

We think Nard had ALS some time before he was diagnosed. His speech was starting to slur. His muscles weren't working as they should. We knew something was seriously wrong. In the months before he passed, the VA provided a specialized van and wheelchair for Nard – as he was a veteran.

Until he died, Nard was always in charge of his health care. If there was anything he specifically needed, Pat made sure it happened. Pat's only focus was on being his caretaker. It was **never** inconvenient for Pat—anything he wanted. Renovation on their home to make it wheelchair accessible were underway.

When he couldn't speak clearly anymore, a device called a Tobii helped. He could type in a message and the Tobii would say it. The Tobii can even communicate simply through eye-tracking technology.

When the end was near, one of Nard's sisters, a physician's assistant, had flown in from Portland to be there for Pat. Mary Kay was there to help, as well. With the new Covid-19 rules both couldn't be in the hospital room simultaneously, so they took turns. It was important for one of them to be there for Pat – not only Nard's wife but the person who really was a sister in every sense of the word. Their sons flew in, and it was very peaceful as they played his favorite music in his room.

Mary Kay shared that just a few hours before death Nard had, what some would describe, as a rally. He opened his eyes, asked for his Tobii, and typed, "How much time to I have?" Pat gave a brilliant, movie-worthy response, "As long as you want." That single sentence describes the love and person that Pat is.

Nard was a quiet Christian. It was important for him to get married in a Catholic church and receive the final sacraments, anointing of the sick and a funeral mass.

I thought back to the question Nard asked Pat and got part of the answer for my question on what someone does when they know death imminent. They are very aware. They know they are at death's door.

Son, Chris, read the eulogy. So beautifully written. So well given. A tough service—but one of celebration thinking about the man named Nard. Burnie. Bunz. Bill.

Nard was born on All Saints Day. Pat had remarked, "Wouldn't it be apropos if Nard made it to April Fool's Day." He was neither saint nor fool. He passed early morning on April first.

But his isn't a story about how he died. This is a message of how the two of them lived. They have two sons, Michael, and Chris. Michael and his wife have three kids: a daughter, Hailey, now in her early twenties, and twin boys in their late teens, Brennan, and Brayden.

Pat is an amazing woman. She took great care of him. Their love affair over the past five decades was amazing. They were married 46 years and together for 48 years. Mary Kay describes them as "crazy nuts about each other." Both lived in Las Vegas when young and met at one of the casinos where Pat waitressed.

You might picture Nard and Pat as one of the original hippies. Pat had never seen him without a beard! Yet, he graduated college, worked for, and retired from, the U.S. Forest Service after 30 years. So did Pat. Whenever Nard got promoted it entailed a move. Regardless of Pat's position with the Forestry Department it always meant that she would need to take a lesser position wherever they moved to help his career. His expertise was determining what trees should be cut down in a forest for logging purposes and to aid the growth of the forest.

It seems to me that true success in a marriage is best described from a movie line in Forest Gump, "they are like peas and carrots." Different, but go perfectly together. That was Nard and Pat.

Music has always been a part of their life. Their first date was a Santana concert. The night of their wedding they went to a Doobie Brothers concert. Mary Kay remembers it well because they took her with them!

They truly were peas and carrots.

On May 30, 1996, a young lady wrote to Dear Abby telling her about someone who took her in when she ran away as a teenager traveling in Las Vegas – where Nard and Pat both lived. It was 1974. Nard and Pat took the runaway in, fed her, and encouraged her to call her folks. They showed her an article Dear Abby had written introducing "Operation Peace of Mind" that allowed kids to communicate with their families that would lead to reuniting them. She had no idea what that person's real name was who took her in. Only knew him as "Nard."

One of Mary Kay's sisters read the article in Dear Abby and realized it was her brother. You can read the actual letter in the picture section of <u>Diagnosed.</u>

Nard and Pat never told anyone about helping the girl. Typical of them both. Years later, when I met my father-in-law for the first time, it was one of the first stories he told me about his son – who was just twenty-one when that happened.

In his last year, Nard was falling frequently, and Pat couldn't get him to his feet. His physical therapist mentioned they could get a pole installed in the house which he could use to pull himself up, as his legs were losing all their strength. Nard asked the therapist if the pole included a dancer.

At one point Nard said to Pat that he thought he was losing his dignity. Her reply was, "Honey, we've been married a long time. You never had any dignity." Their dance. Their love.

One of the things I loved most about Nard was his sense of humor. Until the end that creative, fun side never left. Family parties? He was always at the kids' table having fun with them. His t-shirts always brought smiles to the staff at the ALS center he went to monthly.

At our wedding in 2007, we had one of our nieces take pictures of each couple attending, taped them into a wedding book, and had the guests write a message. Theirs was the best – "Here for the dentists' convention and saw free drinks. Seems like lots of genuinely nice people here."

Classic.

As the three grandkids grew up, they spent a lot of time with Pat and Nard. At least a week in the spring and another week in the autumn. Where they lived in West Virginia at the time was a long drive to where Michael was stationed in the Navy.

When Nard was building a porch, he gave each of his preschool-aged grandsons a tape measure. They measured everything, without comprehending what the numbers meant they just told their grandpa, "It's 13-18." Those boys helped grandpa build the porch. A couple of weeks' job turned into a couple of months with their help.

Haley would pick up rocks and give them to Grandpa and explain to him how each rock used to be a turtle. They would then have a conversation about it for the next half hour.

That was Grandpa. That was Nard.

As a result of treasured times like these, all three grandkids were close to Grandpa and Grandma.

In October, just six months before Nard passed, the family gathered for Nard and MK's father's celebration of life. Their mom passed exactly eight months before Dad. The celebration was in Las Vegas, where the two of them lived after retirement from the Navy. They lived there for decades. The celebration was at their old home—now owned by one of their grandsons (Nard and MK's nephew).

Las Vegas is 1100 miles from Nard and Pat's house in Washington. Nard's son, Michael, wanted his dad to camp with him all the way back. Both knew it would be their final camping trip together. What they didn't plan on was the bitter cold. They managed two nights under the stars before they continued the trip staying in warm hotels. It was an amazing bonding experience for them both.

By this time Nard could barely walk, could hardly talk, and used a breathing machine; but their trip together was perfect.

When they did have to fly somewhere, Alaska Airlines came to the rescue. They couldn't have been any nicer or more accommodating. Pat told them Nard's issues and they provided more than Pat ever would have imagined. In this day of travel complaints, it's nice to know there are people who still jump through hoops for customers.

Mary Kay talked to Pat often during the past couple of years to see how she was doing. Going through something like this affects one's spouse as much as it affects the patient.

Something many forget.

Nard was Mary Kay's only brother. After Mary Kay, four more girls followed in the family's birth order. He was all his sisters' favorite sibling. A true big brother, regardless of their age differences.

Nard taught me how to be a better grandfather. I remember him teaching his three grandkids how to jump inside of an elevator just before it arrived on the floor where they were going. It was all about having fun. He was the nephews and nieces' favorite uncle. There are pictures of him teaching the kids how to make a "Monkey Face."

Nard's high school-aged grandsons called him regularly and talked with him for 45 minutes – even though he was difficult to understand due to ALS. How many high school seniors have that type of relationship with their grandparents? At Mary Kay's parents' celebration of life, just six months ago, I saw his 21-year-old granddaughter wrap her arms around him and sit next to him. She realized how bad he was. She realized this was one of the final times she would have the opportunity to be with him.

Nard taught me how to be a better father by watching his style. His love for his boys. He truly was my brother. In some areas of life, he was my mentor though we weren't even a year apart in age.

From a selfish standpoint we all wanted Nard to be immortal – to be part of our lives, in person, forever. But everyone wanted his suffering to be over. For him to be able to eat. To walk. To breathe.

For Christians throughout the world death is simply the ultimate step to eternity. It doesn't mean, though, that it replaces fear or wonderment. Especially the sadness.

At Nard's celebration of life, the Nard stories flowed. Laughter filled the air. Along with tears of love. Nard impacted everyone he touched. A free spirit without an enemy in the world. A brother, a grandpa, an uncle, a cousin, and a friend who touched everyone he ever met and left them with a smile. What a fantastic way to have a life.

I hope he finds that dentist convention when he gets to heaven.

Case #9:

Marti - Single Mastectomy & Possible Lung Cancer

Getting a personal diagnosis is a very scary event. What is even worse is getting this diagnosis about a family member—especially about a sibling.

It happened for MK about seven years ago—then repeated itself over Thanksgiving, 2022. Both times it was about her sister, Marti. MK was the oldest in a line of five girls. This news was about MK's next oldest sister.

The first time was about breast cancer. More recently, Marti called me and asked me to tell MK about the diagnosis Marti received on Thanksgiving morning from her pulmonologist—lung cancer. I was awaiting a biopsy in just a couple of days for the same issue.

M arti got her annual mammogram about seven years ago. Her internist made sure she scheduled her mammogram in the fall. By the time Marti went, however, it was spring. Great news: her internist called and said nothing to worry about.

Then she got a call from the radiologist. She asked Marti to go back in for another mammogram and this time a sonogram. Her next call was from her internist—the same one who'd said "nothing to worry about"—and who is now her **former** internist. The internist very matter-of-factly said, "You might want to see a breast surgeon" and then just read Marti a list of breast surgeons.

What?!

Why would she need to see a breast surgeon if there was "nothing to worry about"?

Marti went to the breast surgeon, who looked at both the mammogram and sonogram and told Marti it looked like invasive carcinoma and that she recommended a biopsy. She concluded with quite the comment: "Don't worry, you aren't going to die in a month."

When she got home (or probably when she got in the car with husband, Steve), she looked up *invasive carcinoma* and found that is a pretty word for stage III **cancer.**

She needed an oncologist. The breast surgeon lined one up, as well as a plastic surgeon. Fortunately, the breast surgeon did all the heavy lifting. Even showed Marti and Steve pictures and diagrams on the wall describing Marti's case and detailed recommended treatment.

The first thing Marti did was a DNA test for the BRCA gene. It was negative—she was not predisposed to breast cancer.

A lumpectomy was out of the question as she had cancer, which made that invasive carcinoma, in seven lymph nodes.

Marti and Steve learned that there had been signs that should have indicated there was an issue. But when one isn't looking for breast cancer signs, one doesn't see them—even if they are obvious to trained eyes.

Marti chose a single mastectomy instead of a double mastectomy. Her chances of getting breast cancer were 1 in 8. Getting cancer in the other breast carried the same odds—the odds didn't increase simply because she had cancer in the other breast.

Marti and Steve had to tell their two adult kids. And their parents. The way Marti and Steve presented it was not a life changer for the kids: they explained that the cancer wasn't life-ending, just life-changing. For MK and Marti's mom it was easy: "Welcome to the club," Mom said. She already was a survivor of a couple of diverse kinds of cancer.

It was quite different for Steve's mom. Steve's sister had died of breast cancer years before when she was in her early thirties.

Mastectomy. Chemo. Then radiation. The process would be simple.

Marti was fifty-nine. She got her diagnosis in May, surgery in July, then chemo in September over a 12-week period.

After her mastectomy, the plastic surgeon inserted a spacer. The breast reconstruction completion would take place much later, after the chemo and radiation treatments.

Chemo would be simple. Every two weeks for the first four sessions. Then once a week for the next eight. Marti lost her hair before the second treatment. Both Marti and MK remember that it came back very curly! Never was before. Marti would continue working and would get her chemo late afternoon on Thursday. Then she would have the weekend to recuperate in bed.

The best thing about chemo was her "posse": two other women going through the same thing, just a week or two behind Marti in the process. They became friends and are still friends today.

Marti remembers the process like yesterday. Arrive with her snacks and a special blanket to keep her warm, get a strong dose of Benadryl to help her sleep. Then a steroid. Then the specially mixed chemo—based on her blood counts when she arrived.

Her new friends, Pauline and Krista also had breast cancer. Pauline and Marti were just a year apart in age. Krista was thirty. The three would jabber about anything and everything while they were there. Laughter filled the room. Steve remembers that all three would sleep through their treatments. Like clockwork.

All three lost their tastebuds differently. Marti's snacks always had to be spicy. Pauline loved muffins and Krista loved extremely sweet snacks.

They attended the bell-ringing ceremony for each other, gifting each other a token that is still incredibly special to this day. They talk with each other often on Facebook. Marti talks about the support that she got from family and these two new friends as extremely important in her process.

In retrospect Marti would have had a double mastectomy because of the follow-up required. She must go in every six months for a 4D mammogram of her healthy breast as well as a chest X-ray and MRI – all to make sure she doesn't get cancer in that breast. If she had had a double at the same time, this process wouldn't be necessary.

Fast forward several years to 2021. Marti had no issues. She was still working at the same company where she had worked for almost 20 years. She was feeling fine.

But later in the year, she began getting stomach pains. Back to the hospital for a colonoscopy, endoscopy, and an ERCP that threaded a camera down her throat to look for problems in the liver, gallbladder, bile ducts, and pancreas. They found that Marti had polyps in the duodenum. In most cases, as it would be with Marti, the polyps were benign but needed to be removed as they have a malignant potential.

January 2022. Full abdominal surgery to cut out the polyps. Success. Six months later, they came back and were, again, growing on the duodenum. More surgery in November. This time the doctors found that her gall bladder was inflamed and opted to remove it. They removed her duodenum as well.

Four weeks later she started having pancreatitis. It became so bad Steve rushed her to the hospital to see if it could be calmed down. She couldn't eat anything and was weak.

Thanksgiving morning. Still in the hospital. MK and I had spent Thanksgivings with Marti, Steve, and the kids—but never in the hospital. Our phone rang. It was Marti asking to talk with me. We thought it was simply to find out how I was doing awaiting my own biopsy for lung cancer.

She tells me her pulmonologist had just left her hospital room after giving her jarring news. She has . . . . lung cancer! Same diagnosis as me. She wants me to tell her sister as she knows that MK knows how to deal with this after 20 days of waiting for my biopsy. (This was Day 22 of my own journey.)

MK heard our conversation and jumped on the phone. Marti's hospital was less than two hours from our house. MK asked if we could come over and spend Thanksgiving with her and Steve—sans turkey!

For the next few weeks Mary Kay and Marti talked regularly. She finally got out of the hospital, talked to her oncologist from her breast surgery, and got a biopsy scheduled. We waited, anxiously, for the results. By this time, we'd received the wonderful news on my biopsy results.

Marti's biopsy comes back with great news, too: she doesn't have cancer in her liver!

Wait— what?

The biopsy was supposed to be for a mass in the **lung**—not the liver!

It would be weeks later when Marti and Steve learned what was happening inside her body. Her liver was now pushing up on her lung. The mass in her CT scan wasn't a mass at all—it was her liver, explaining how the liver was biopsied.

GREAT news! She is still cancer-free!

When we spent a weekend with Marti and Steve recently, I had a chance to ask Steve what it was like for him standing by Marti through all this.

Steve said it was very tough. There was nothing he could do. Very tough for a business owner who is relied upon daily to make all the decisions and figure out how to get things done and customers taken care of regardless of personal issues.

They've been married 41 years and are remarkably close! He looks forward to retirement and spending their sixties enjoying life. His mom is ninety-seven. Marti and MK's parents lived into their nineties. Genetics told both they had years go enjoy life together. They've been dating since their teens when they met at work at McDonalds. Life-long sweethearts looking forward to the golden years.

Steve said he had several friends to get him through the tough times.

Marti has always been a glass-half-full person. The more rain, the fuller the glass gets. It was always a matter of "when I am 100%," not "if I am ever 100% again." She was never worried.

Her prayers didn't change. She'd thank God for getting her through today and tell Him she'd reach out to Him tomorrow and thank Him, again, for getting her that day as well.

Before the 2021 surgery Steve and Marti had already purchased a large RV. Another one of MK and Marti's sisters has one—but they live on the West coast. Their goal was to meet each other halfway across the United States, both in their RVs, and spend family time together. MK and I will fly out to meet them and celebrate!

Case #10:

Nancy-Lung Cancer

I met Nancy, The Telephone Doctor, as we were using one of her services at our company many years ago. Once you meet her you are instantly a fan of hers for life. Her smile is infectious! She has authored several books. Every time I read one of them, I sit back and say, "Duh, I should have thought of that." Mary Kay and I have had dinner with Nancy and husband, Dick. They are now good friends. I'm still her biggest fan. I've seen her present at a convention. Magnetizing. Everyone I've ever referred to is so glad I did so.
Recently I heard the rest of her story. She introduces what happened to her as, "COVID Saved My Life."

When COVID hit, Nancy and Dick decided to stop going to their gym. They loved going there and had been going to the same gym faithfully for 17 years.

It was an easy decision. Due to COVID the gym was forced to close temporarily.

It's a boutique, locally owned gym: Fitness Edge in St. Louis. Owned by a former Mr. St. Louis, Mr. Missouri, and first runner-up in a Mr. America Competition—who was also a friend of the family.

Luckily, they had a home gym that was being used as anything but a gym. They now had to use it for what it was. It was well appointed for anything they might need. Nancy whispered quietly to me, "I never used Suzanne Somers's thigh machine. Please don't tell her—it's a bitch to use." That's Nancy!

For a few weeks during COVID, they had their trainer from Fitness Edge come to the house. The trainer helped them understand how to use all the equipment properly. Their home workouts were so different than the time they spent at the gym, but they both were happy they were working out.

One day in early August, Nancy used the health rider ab machine differently. Thinking she was still 35 years old; she did the exercise slowly: she pulled in very, very slowly and then let go in an extremely slow motion. She was convinced this would strengthen her core and she would look great in front a 3,000-person audience. She still isn't sure it helped her core, but she did hurt her ribcage muscles.

A week after Nancy did that exercise, she experienced the most uncomfortable sensation she'd ever felt in the ribcage area. She knew she had better see the doctor.

After hearing her story, the doctor agreed that she must have pulled something. His prescription was to give it time, take a break from the machine, and then do a CT scan.

A week later she returned to the doctor. This time she asked for a CT scan because the muscle aches were not subsiding.

The doctor ordered a CT scan of Nancy's abdomen and pelvis. The doctor told her they found gallstones, which would not cause the muscle issue, then continued": "You can live with this. We'll do another CT scan in 30 days."

The next week, Dick had a doctor appointment for allergies. After their doctor was done with Dick's appointment, Nancy casually mentioned the muscle issue that had been there around about a month. The doctor knew that she had already had a CT scan but thought they should do a chest X-ray while she was there. The CT scan didn't cover the chest area.

The next day the doctor called. The chest X-ray showed a small abnormal nodule on her right lung. Three days later she had outpatient surgery to take a biopsy of the nodule. Quick. No pain.

Frankly, Nancy was more nervous of the mandatory COVID-19 test that was given in the hospital garage before she could do the surgery. Great news. No COVID.

She had a choice of the hospital and surgeon she would use. One was a young doctor who knew all the latest procedures. She chose the doc in his mid-seventies. For those of us who are retired, he was a Marcus Welby type of doctor, but without the bedside manner. Before Nancy went in for surgery she told the doctor, "You can't operate on me today unless you smile and are in a good mood." She waited until he did!

The surgery wasn't painful. She was up and doing a lap around the hospital wing the next day. Two laps the day after that, then three. Turned out the small mass in her right lobe was cancerous but no lymph glands were affected.

Nancy realized she was richly blessed. If it hadn't been for COVID, she and Dick would have still been going to Fitness Edge. She wouldn't have been exercising at home with an ab machine. She wouldn't have used the ab machine improperly, and she may have never strained her ribcage muscles.

She attributes the quick healing to a couple of things. Nancy is **always** positive. Her mother, Esther, taught her, *"It is never the problem—it is how you handle it."* Nancy has taught her grandkids this already. Well, that blows her cover. She is *not* thirty-five anymore.

She had COVID masks created that have a huge smile on them. Mary Kay and I wore them to a concert, so we know those masks bring huge smiles.

Nancy has, as she describes, her own great relationship with God. The cancer didn't bring out more prayers. Faith is part of her life. She prays every morning. She is grateful for life and the blessings the two of them have experienced in life—and always will be.

This little thing called cancer was not about to change her outlook and attitude.

Case #11:

Vicki–Breast Cancer & a Lumpectomy

I went to high school with Vicki and her cousins. We lived on the same street—about five houses apart. We both attended our 50th high school reunion last September.

Had no idea she spent her first two years teaching at the same Lutheran grade school where I attended through eighth grade. Had no idea she went to a sister church of St. Paul's, across town. The school I played football and basketball against in 6th and 8th grade.

Most importantly, I didn't know her amazing story. Enjoy and learn.

I t was May 2003. Vicki was with her dad at a hospital in Madison, Wisconsin, about sixty miles away from where we grew up, when he got the news that he had a rare form of colon cancer. She had been in the health care field for years and thought she might help.

A month after her dad was diagnosed, Vicki found a lump on her breast. Her doctor, whom she had seen for the past 15 years and worked with in the medical field, suggested she get a mammogram. She did. The doctor ordered a biopsy.

Waiting for the biopsy—then the results—was nerve-racking. When the doctor called, he said he wanted to see her that day. Since her husband was working out of town for the day, she went alone and learned that she had cancer. She needed to see a surgeon.

It was tough letting the kids and her parents know. She remembers at one point sitting on the steps and crying. Her daughter, home from college, sat down and put her arms around her, saying, "Don't worry, Mom. We'll go wig shopping."

Her surgeon recommended a lumpectomy. Mastectomies weren't common back then. After the lumpectomy would be chemo. In January would be radiation.

She waited for the lumpectomy from the 14th of June until the 23rd of July. After the surgery she took a week off. It was the only extended time she took off through chemo and radiation!

She continued trying to go with her dad to his cancer appointments to support him, as well as her mom, emotionally. Vicki started her own chemo treatments right after Labor Day. She had twelve sessions, with a two-week break between each.

In October 2003, her dad had a heart attack and died instantly. Vicki still wonders if his chemo treatment was the cause; it just took so much out of him.

Mom now focused on being there for Vicki. Chemo was tough. It made Vicki sick. Today she still remembers her aversion to certain smells during treatment and still sometimes gets nauseated by them.

She scheduled her chemo treatments on Thursday or Friday afternoons. She could take a day of vacation if it were Thursday afternoon to recover on Friday. For Friday chemo sessions she had the weekend to recover.

Radiation started in January 2004 and lasted six weeks, five days a week. Treatment took about 45 minutes, from start to finish. Her body would either be tattooed for the sessions, or she could use a magic marker to mark where the radiation needed to be. She opted for the marker and redrew the lines each time after she showered.

Vicki entered remission and she returned to her precancer life.

In 2011 Vicki's mom got kidney cancer. Mom had a kidney removed. And in 2012, Mom started chemo. Fortunately, Mom had the same oncologist as Vicki. During one of Mom's visits, the oncologist told Vicki that he was "kicking her out now." She had been cancer-free for nearly 10 years! Sadly, in January 2013, Mom died. The year before she felt great, was walking every day and feeling better than she had in a long time. The chemo, however, took its toll on her, as it had Vicki's dad.

Vicki knew what chemo could do. Although she didn't take any sick days, she remembers days at her office and using the waste basket under her desk for something besides papers.

Five years ago, Vicki's brother, Jim, was diagnosed with breast cancer. He got a double mastectomy. His was the first male case I've personally known of.

The siblings took the BRCA test. I'm very aware of this because Mary Kay's mom, who died from cervical cancer, took the same test, and found she was negative—so MK and her four sisters didn't worry about it.

The BRCA gene test is a blood test that uses DNA analysis to identify harmful changes (mutations) in either one of the two breast cancer susceptibility genes — BRCA1 and BRCA2.

People who inherit mutations in these genes are at an increased risk of developing breast cancer and ovarian cancer compared with the general population.

The BRCA gene test is offered to those who are likely to have an inherited mutation based on personal or family history of breast cancer or ovarian cancer. The BRCA gene test isn't routinely performed on people at average risk of breast and ovarian cancers.

The results of genetic testing aren't always clear. A positive result means you carry a gene mutation that increases your risk of cancer, and you can work with your doctor to manage that risk. A negative result may mean that you don't have the mutation or that you might have a gene mutation doctors haven't discovered yet. Your test might also identify a gene variant that doctors aren't certain about. In these situations, it's not always clear what the results mean for your cancer risk.

Most people considering genetic testing undergo genetic counseling. Genetic counseling can help you understand what the results could mean for your health, help you decide whether genetic testing is right for you, and recommend a specific set of genetic tests based on your family history.

Based on results, one may choose to have a mastectomy, as Angelina Jolie chose very publicly, or may choose extra vigilant monitoring of your body.

Vicki told me her personal faith, the support she received from her husband and her kids helped her through her trial. Oh, and prayer.

Prayer. Both of her doctors asked, "Can I pray with you?" Both did—which calmed her. She now believes that the power of prayer was instrumental in her healing and her continued health.

Her pastor gave her a book of prayers, which she has paid forward to other cancer patients by giving that same book to them when they had issues.

It was a blessing talking to someone I knew so well who faced cancer herself, as well as with her mom, dad, and brother. She and her brother are still here to talk about their journey!

Robert-Prostate Cancer

*Mary Kay and I know Robert and his wife, Kitty. We worked
with him, we have been to their house, we looked forward to
the Christian books that the two of them would provide for
everyone at our office at Christmas – every year.*
*Robert was the President of Glass Doctor, years before I took
the helm. I loved the relationship he had with so many of our
franchisees. Some traveled with him and even stayed at his
home when visiting headquarters in Waco.*
*Another close friend of ours went on retreats with Robert at
their Catholic church. Robert knew that this would be his
God-given mission on retirement.*

Robert was a real health nut. He exercised at least five days a week.
Strenuously. He was one of the fastest walkers I've ever seen in my
life—the type of walker I couldn't keep up with even when jogging.

It was a regular appointment with his family doctor that started all of
this. Because of Robert's age, the doctor thought they should check Roberts
PSA—normal stuff when a man turns fifty. The PSA came up a few points
high. So, the doctor thought they should keep a close eye on it.

Just before Martin Luther King Day 2010, his doctor decided they
should conduct a biopsy. Robert wasn't worried—no cancer in his family
and 75% of the men diagnosed with prostate cancer were sixty-five and older.
He was only just over fifty!

The biopsy showed cancer. His Gleason score was six, which means the tumor was less aggressive and more likely to grow more slowly. Still, it was cancer. He called his wife, Kitty, and gave her the news.

Robert couldn't talk to anyone else right away. Stunned into silence—which is tough for someone with Robert's personality! He gave this problem to God.

Quite different from 10 years prior. Robert was in Las Vegas delivering a speech and a weird experience startled him. As he lay in bed one evening Robert saw a message on the ceiling: just the word "Robert." Immediately his body started to shake violently. No idea why!

While still in Vegas, he went to a magic shop at Caesar's Palace to buy something for his boys. While there he noticed an art gallery with a picture, he thought would be ideal for his office. Suddenly he heard the words in his head, "You can't spend the money for this—it is God's money."

Upon his return home from Las Vegas, Robert heard from his office manager that she and her husband had visited a church that weekend that she thought Robert might enjoy.

He hadn't attended church before this. He didn't have a relationship with Jesus. He visited the church and enjoyed the service. He returned once but was left unfulfilled because it wasn't a spiritual experience for him.

The assistant pastor of the church invited him to a newcomer's class. Robert can still picture that day—walking into a room that seemed pitch black. A light came to convince him he had lived the first 40 years of his life backwards. Focused only on money, nothing else. Robert knew that he needed to change—immediately!

As Robert was talking to a close friend, the friend remarked that Robert was different. Robert shared his newfound faith with his friend, who then told Robert about a speaker coming to Waco. This man was Patrick Morley, who wrote *Man in the Mirror*. (Mary Kay and I saw Patrick speak almost 20 years later.)

That same night Robert saw Patrick speak, God put two things in Robert's mind and heart:

Take a Man in the Mirror class in Waco.

Create a Bible study for Catholic men.

Robert wasn't even Catholic at that point. This was a curious message at the time. When he met Kitty in 1999, he hadn't even worshipped in a Catholic church. Fortunately, she was a cradle Catholic.

He started a Bible study for members of his church and their friends. When he joined Kitty in her Catholic church, he expanded the study to include men in her parish. It was a hit. Soon he hosted a weekend retreat in his home. It was then the priest discovered that he wasn't even a Catholic.

Robert attended classes one night a week for three hours to learn the Bible. His questions answered, Robert and Kitty have worshipped together in their Catholic church since then.

Fast forward to 2010 as he faced cancer diagnosis.

The weekend after the diagnosis Robert and Kitty researched prostate cancer. He had a tough time finding anyone under the age of sixty to talk to about this. Had a bunch of questions for Monday morning, though, when he started calling people and doctors.

Monday was MLK Day. Everything was closed. All he could think of was "when people make plans, God just laughs." Through their research he discovered the best solution for someone his age was to remove the cancer with Da Vinci surgery—a robotic surgical system that uses a minimally invasive approach. Robert learned that if you don't surgically remove the cancer and simply choose radiation, that it might come back and, as he phrased it, you would become toast!

One major problem: Robert lived in Waco, Texas. No one in Waco performed this surgery.

A solution-finder, not a problem-finder, Robert started looking in Dallas, less than two hours north of Waco. He produced twenty-one questions he would ask the doctors he interviewed who used this type of surgery. It came down to two doctors for their final decision on who to use for surgery.

His final question of both doctors was "Are you a prayerfully Godly man?" Only one of them gave the answer Robert and Kitty wanted. A doctor who replied that he had his prayer journal in his pocket—then showed it to them. Decision made. Robert gave the doctor a Saint Peregrine (the patron saint of cancer sufferers) medal.

The surgery was March 1, 2010.

Robert remembers being at mass after the surgery with tears running down his face. Tears of joy that he was still alive. If he hadn't survived, he would have been in heaven. But he was ready to make lifestyle changes and genuinely enjoy his wonderful marriage.

Robert decided to take all seven weeks of vacation he had earned. He was in a key role at work, but he had a blessing of life. He would change his workaholic ways.

That was over thirteen years ago. How life has changed since then.

Robert leads the Central Texas Catholic Men's Conference. In March of 2023 they will have their 11th conference. Robert and Kitty had a vision of Robert creating a men's ministry program for the Austin Diocese. They shared this with the Bishop of the Austin Diocese at dinner one evening.

His retirement in 2019 has allowed his full-time commitment for the Lord's work. Robert started a Catholic men's leaders' organization, the Catholic Men's Leadership Alliance. Although he donates his time, he has five staff members who operate the organization.

It has been 13 years since prostate cancer and still no complications. No chemo. No radiation. No scares.

Robert knows that men are different. We think we can control things. We believe that we can even control cancer if it happens to us. We can't. All we can do is control what happens in our lives after we receive the biggest scare of our lives—and make sure we give it to God!

Case #13:

Pam–DES & Cervical Cancer

Pam, Mary Kay, and I all worked together over fifteen years ago. We've lost track over time but know each other well as our offices are just feet from each other. Usually, Pam and I were in the same meetings, but didn't know about personal issues.

P am was born in the 1960s. When her mom was pregnant with her, she took a drug to help prevent a miscarriage. It wasn't until Pam read the article that she learned something difficult for her to hear.

The following is a *Time* magazine article from March 24, 1980. The article starts like this:

DES DAUGHTERS

Some two million pregnant women had taken DES (diethylstilbestrol) to help prevent miscarriage before the Food and Drug Administration alerted physicians to its dangers in 1971. Doctors suspected that the estrogen drug was causing vaginal and cervical cancer in daughters born to those women, and more recently have also implicated it in genital abnormalities and infertility in sons. Now there is more unsettling news for DES daughters. When they reach childbearing age, they appear to be more vulnerable than others to miscarriage—as well as to stillbirth, premature birth, and ectopic pregnancy (in which the fetus grows outside the uterus).

Pam found other sources that identified this drug as causing a tilted uterus and maybe even affecting the brain.

Pam's first pregnancy: an ectopic pregnancy.

This pregnancy almost killed her. She rushed to the hospital as she was bleeding profusely. Seven pints of blood were standing by. In surgery she was given anticoagulants to stop the bleeding. Very painful.

She contracted cervical cancer when she was just twenty-nine. She didn't know why these things were happening to her. The article hadn't been written yet.

She got through this time by crying a great deal. She learned that when terrible things happen, you simply must pivot and keep going.

Three pregnancies followed. So did three more miscarriages. At her doctor's insistence, she had a hysterectomy. This was a tough decision because she really wanted kids.

Pivot. Pam decided that she and her husband should consider adoption. Her husband at the time was, at the time, dead set against this.

Pam was in her forties when she read a *Time* magazine article about DES. Pam learned for the first time what was happening to her body and why!

Her next medical challenge was with freckles. Pam had had them since she was a kid. Being from Florida it was "the thing" to lie in the sun and get tan. She never considered what might happen years later as a result.

In 2010 she got melanoma and needed Mohs surgery.

This surgery required a lab set up next to the operating table. Every time the doctor removed a layer of skin, the technician examined it for cancer. They kept cutting until Pam was cancer-free in the area. If you met her, you might notice the big divot in her leg from surgery.

The day after surgery, her brother died.

More pivots—but keep on going.

Twice more she had melanoma, but both were in the preliminary stages. The only surgeries needed were completed in the doctor's office.

Most recently Pam had a bandage on her arm from squamous cell carcinoma. It gets "cut out" without going too deep.

Pam's dad, a physician, died of squamous cell carcinoma. Even though he had been treated for these cancers several times, he waited too long, and the cancer metastasized in his brain.

Today she feels great. She is active but is now smart enough to not expose any areas to the sun. She says she got through it all with the support of family and friends.

Amazing how a medicine that her mom took so long ago that was designed to ensure her life nearly took it. Pam is jaded but knows that whatever life gives her, she will simply pivot. Then she'll take on the next challenge.

Case #14:

Sue-Throat Cancer

I worked for Sue's two brothers, Bob, and Bill, in the mid-'80s. Still great friends. Saw them both last summer. Last spring MK I and stayed at Bob's house in Georgia as we were traveling south to Florida. Sue was staying with him. Had a great night playing Mexican Train. This past spring the two of them stayed at our condominium in Florida. Again, wonderful time. Here we are almost 40 years later. I knew Sue but I never knew her story. Goes back to we never know what anyone is going through at any given time. Can't wait until they visit us this summer. We'll hug her tighter than we ever did before.
(Note: Names are changed in this article per their request.)

If you live in Buffalo, New York, you understand it is going to snow ... a lot. You also live in a football town where most people know that Jim Kelly is one of the greatest quarterbacks in history and is now a member of the Pro Football Hall of Fame. Residents like Sue also know Jim Kelly's story about his fight with squamous cell carcinoma.

Usually around Christmastime Sue would be worn down and inevitably end up with a sore throat, laryngitis, and a bad cold. Sometimes the doctor would give her an antibiotic, which usually cleared things up. In fall of 2012 she was headed on a cruise. Same symptoms. Called the doctor, got the antibiotic, and went on the cruise.

Fall of 2013, she still had same symptoms off and on, but doctors didn't think it was anything. Eventually she was referred to an ear, nose, and throat doctor. He performed tests but wrote symptoms off to acid reflux or stomach issues and sent her on her way. She even visited an osteopath for treatments, as well as a physical therapist for neck massages and treatments.

As she was prepping for her daughter Jen's August wedding, she had little time to worry about her ongoing discomfort as it still had not improved much. No real pain or aggravation, just more annoyance than anything else. Sue had a busy life and didn't have time to focus on a sore throat.

During that summer of 2014, she repeated her symptoms to her GP, and mentioned that having seen news articles about Jim Kelly's cancer symptoms, as well as the symptoms of well-known Buffalo Sabres' sportscaster Rick Jeanerette, she'd realized "those are the same symptoms I have!"

She was referred to Kelly's doctors, who, after the initial consultation, ordered scans and an endoscopy. Both showed a mass in her throat. She still had two more weddings to go to in September, so she postponed doing a biopsy until her return. She still remembers her doctor saying, with a smile, "Well, when your social calendar settles down, let's get you in here." She'd already waited two years for "something" to show up, so what was another two weeks!

The biopsy resulted in a diagnosis of throat cancer in October 2014. They explained that this was due to the HPV virus. Most HPV infections don't lead to cancer, but cancer in the back of the throat (oropharyngeal) has been linked to HPV infection. The good news was that it was curable.

Sue's doctors gave her a step-by-step list of what to expect and when. They also gave recommendations for further care. She met with the chemo people, the radiation people, the dental people, and the "feeding tube" people. The doctors' input was perfect.

She did more due diligence and consulted with other treatment centers and doctors. Her sister went with her to make sure the notes they took were complete. Between doctors and family and friends she gained a complete understanding of what was about to happen.

The doctors told her she would eventually lose the ability to swallow. She did. They told her she would lose her sense of taste. She did. The food tasted awful. Even her favorite wine would taste like paste. She eventually wouldn't be able to eat at all. Throat swells, esophageal muscles don't work so well, epiglottis forgets what to do! Smoothies might help—for a while.

Sue was scheduled to have a feeding tube into her stomach for nutrition. A feeding bag that, midway through her radiation treatments, had to be changed three times a day, till she could eat by mouth again, was uncomfortable, but preferable. Every 30 seconds it would shoot food/nutrition into her stomach as she could no longer eat.

She would need a dose of chemo. This would get her cells ready for six and a half weeks of radiation. The chemo sessions would last six hours. She would have two more chemo sessions: one in the middle of the radiation treatment cycle, and one at the end, if warranted. Fortunately, she had none of the side effects usually associated with chemo.

Next, she would have dry mouth (and still does), as well as tons of mucus in her nose and throat being produced to offset the dry mouth problem.

Next, exhaustion.

Buffalo suffered from "Snowvember" on days three through five of Sue's beginning radiation week! Driving ban as roads are closed. She would be delayed a couple of days.

The radiation would take its toll and she would be weak. A fentanyl transdermal patch would dispense pain medicine. She remembers hearing from Jen and her sisters Barbara and Tammy about the hallucinations she had during that time.

To prepare for the radiation, prior to the actual regimen of treatments, material that felt like a warm facecloth was put on her face. It had holes through it, especially around the eyes, mouth, and nostrils. In twenty minutes, it had hardened into a mask that looked like something Freddie from Halloween would've worn.

The hardened mask was put over her face and then clipped to the table she was lying on. She finally realized this was part of the process. Next, her body was belted to the table, like seatbelts. She had previously had a PET scan, which showed **exactly** where the cancer was in her throat so the radiation could be properly targeted.

Shortly after radiation was completed, she wanted to go to Cabo San Lucas with Jen and her husband. Her doctor nixed this trip. Mexico isn't well known for their great medical care. Two months after the radiation she asked him if she could make a trip to England in May, where she used to live, to see friends there. Although the doctor wasn't crazy about the idea, he relented because of medical help there is great. She didn't need it.

Dental hygiene was another challenge. Saliva glands produce fluid to break down enzymes to aid digestion, but also provide a type of bacteria that helps fight tooth decay. In her dental appointments since 2015, Sue has routinely had cavities—which was new.

For the next several years, she continued annual checkups. Then in January of 2023 her annual cancer appointment with her doctor in Buffalo was excellent, no issues whatsoever. In the early years she looked at that routine appointment with great trepidation.

Sue talks about the keys to her getting through this time: family, friends, and prayer. She remembers especially her two sisters, her sister-in-law, and her five brothers. Every week or so, she would update all of them about her progress. The responses she got in return made her feel as if they were putting a warm blanket around her. Her daily journal was therapeutic and a way to connect with those that cared about her. She recommends this to others as it was an aid to her progress.

Sue is a huge believer in prayer. Her family is spread around and each encouraged members of their churches pray for her. She said she could feel the prayers. She couldn't emphasize enough how neighbors, family, and friends were so important. Sue has always had strong faith. She doesn't believe that God healed her, specifically, because of her personal prayers. But no one can ever make her believe that prayer doesn't work.

Who would have thought that Jim Kelly could help a fan—in such a hugely unique way. Not because of his throwing arm—but because of his doctors.

Go, BILLS!

Case #15:

Kathy–Her Mom's Ovarian Cancer

I love the "once upon a time" stories that end with "and they lived happily ever after." This is one of those stories.

Mary Kay and I know Kathy, but this story is about her mom. Kathy was a sales manager for one of our franchisees in the Pacific Northwest. MK ran the Los Angeles operation. We've seen Kathy at conventions and meetings but haven't seen her since 2009 when we left that company.

It was great to catch up with her, but it was even better to learn her mom's story.

Kathy was born when her mom was only eighteen. Her parents got divorced when Kathy was ten, and she and her mom have remained remarkably close.

Cancer runs rampant in Kathy's family. Three aunts died of breast cancer and one of lung cancer before Kathy started her own family. Dad has survived prostate cancer twice and duodenum cancer more recently. He is now eighty-five.

Kathy was in college when her mom called to let her know she needed a hysterectomy. Mom was just thirty-six at the time and, while she didn't plan to have more kids, her surgeon left both ovaries intact to let her go through menopause "naturally." Looking back, Mom wished they would have removed them at the same time. But then we wouldn't have a remarkable story that ends with "and everyone lived happily after."

By 1996 Kathy was married and had a seven-year-old and a two-year-old. Mom called with news that she might have fibromyalgia and irritable bowel syndrome. Her local doctor sent her in for a colonoscopy to see if anything else would show up.

Cancer wasn't on the horizon yet, but soon poked its ugly head. The doctor who had performed the colonoscopy admitted her to Northwest Hospital for additional testing. That testing included an ultrasound of her abdomen where ascites (a type of fluid build-up) was found, and the diagnosis became obvious. Doctors wanted to do surgery immediately and as luck would have it, the gynecological surgeon on call that weekend was renowned in the ovarian cancer world!

He came out after surgery and said he was able to get 99% of the cancer. Some were impossible to get, but chemo would take care of that. He was the same doctor who had performed successful ovarian cancer surgery on Kathy's aunt (her mom's next-door neighbor for her adult life), who is now ninety-one.

During this entire time Kathy and her husband were just closing on a larger home, making them able to accommodate Mom during recovery. Her husband installed beautiful French doors that opened to a huge deck on the same floor as mom's room. She could go out and enjoy the weather, and Kathy was still able to nurse her when necessary. She sure enjoyed having her grandchildren right there, too!

To this day Kathy's mom tells everyone that she has the best son-in-law in the world—one who opened their home to her and made her feel so welcome.

Kathy describes her mom as a curvy German/Norwegian woman. The doctor never mentioned her weight as an issue. Instead, the opposite. The doctor told them that some people die of starvation before the cancer kills them. Mom was safe!

Both Kathy and her mom are positive. Almost Pollyanna-ish. They both look at problems simply as challenges to fight together. Yes, she had cancer—but they would attack any issues with cancer together and at least were given the opportunity to fight.

Chemo treatments were mother-daughter time. Kathy went with mom to every appointment and built jigsaw puzzles with her. Afterwards, Kathy would take Mom to Jamba Juice to get something to replenish them both. It helped chemo treatment end on a positive note.

Kathy did research on ovarian cancer and found that if one makes it through five years clear of recurring disease, the chances are great that the person won't get it again.

Mom returned to her home and babysat the kids to give Kathy and her husband a chance to travel more together. The weekend of Kathy's husband's 40th birthday, they went to celebrate in Las Vegas. At this point mom was cancer-free for not two years.

Mom mentioned that she didn't feel great when she arrived to be with the kids but didn't go into detail. Soon she learned the ovarian cancer had returned.

Different hospital, same oncologist, same surgeon. When the doctor came out this time, he shared that it had spread but he got **all** of it, as well as any that had spread. 100% this time.

The oncologist told mom and daughter that he had never had a patient who suffered ovarian cancer twice and beat it. The goal now would be to manage this for as long as possible. Little did the doctor know that mom would still be alive 22 years later!

She moved back into Kathy's house during treatment weeks. It was her home away from home and a beautiful place for her to recuperate.

Kathy noticed petty things that bothered mom. When she lost her hair, nothing was invented yet for the eyebrows. When mom looked in the mirror it was a harsh reminder that she'd had cancer twice.

She left the port in her chest for a year—just in case. She was eager for doctor appointments now. Mom never was comfortable when the appointments went to six months and a year. She needed constant check-in and reminder that all was well.

Now, Mom is a great support to others. Both times she joined online support groups. A woman she met in the group lost her own mom but is now a family member. They exchange Christmas cards, and mom sends her gifts every year. Someday they will even meet.

This journey has shaped and molded Kathy. Because her parents were divorced, she never supported her dad like she did her mom, and she wasn't a part of his daily life. She has always felt bad because of this. During her dad's last round of cancer, she made a point of supporting him and spending more time with him.

Kathy can't imagine anyone going through the ordeal mom did without always having someone with them virtually. Taking notes for the patient is so important to make sure the one going through treatment can listen, and then refer to those notes as it can all become a blur. She is concerned that, left alone, a person will listen to all the things going through their mind by themselves.

Mom is now eighty. Her doctor now has a patient who survived ovarian cancer twice. And they all lived happily ever after.

Case #16:

Bryan-Thyroid Cancer

The last time I saw Bryan was pre-COVID. I was working with the president of a franchise company in Cincinnati. Bryan was a wiz at local marketing for franchisees. After I retired in 2020, I lost track of him—until last week.

When I was there, Bryan's wife, Amanda, had just given birth to Jonah. They were so excited to have that baby boy. His wife ended up in the hospital for 27 days after delivery. The baby was home, and Bryan was doing his best to balance working, going to the hospital, and caring for the baby.

Bryan had a fireplug build, red hair, and a great bushy red beard. As you will see, the beard became part of the challenge for him—about to be revealed.

About Valentine's Day of 2022 Bryan switched jobs. He and Amanda decided that it would be best for the family if they moved closer to other family members, about eighty miles south of Cleveland and 175 miles from Cincy. For the family this was a major move. It required much prayer.

Before the move, Bryan had been focusing on his health. He had dropped forty pounds by cutting back to 1800 calories a day. There came a time, though, that regardless of his 1800-calorie regimen he just wasn't dropping any more weight. Amanda, a nurse, was concerned. The doctor felt that he was fine, but his wife thought there might be a deeper problem. She suggested an ultrasound to see if there were any issues causing this, but the doctor declined.

The move was tough. They prayed and prayed about it, asking for guidance. They were convinced this was the right decision. Bryan went to work for the owner of a startup who was previously a coworker. They were good friends, and the new job was ideal for him.

With the move, the family found a new primary care physician. Bryan believes this alone might have saved his life. When the new PCP heard about Bryan's challenge of losing more weight, she immediately sent him to a specialist, who did an ultrasound. It was revealed that Bryan had tumors on his thyroid. Because of Bryan's huge beard, it was hard to find them on his neck under that beard.

No one had previously asked about the history of thyroid issues in the family. An aunt had had her thyroid removed. His grandfather was found to have thyroid tumors after a postmortem autopsy. The specialist referred Bryan to a surgeon to see whether he should have a biopsy taken or simply undergo surgery. It was obvious that his tumors were large. No one yet knew how large.

Bryan had outpatient surgery. Everyone was surprised when the surgery discovered that one of his tumors was larger than a cell phone. Previous doctors in Cincy said that thyroid issues are uncommon for nonsmoking men.

The tumors were biopsied after surgery. The finding: cancer.

Although the surgery was outpatient, Bryan felt like his arms were on fire when he got home. His wife, being a nurse, knew how to take him immediately to the ER. They found out that his troponin levels were extremely high. According to ClevelandClinic.org:

> A troponin test looks for the protein troponin (there are two forms related to your heart, troponin I and troponin T) in your blood. Normally, troponin stays inside your heart muscle's cells, but damage to those cells — like the kind of damage from a heart attack — causes troponin to leak into your blood. Higher levels of troponin in your blood also mean more heart damage, which can help healthcare providers determine the severity of a heart attack.

Four days later it was finally determined that his heart was OK. The cancer docs decided a total thyroid removal was the right course of action as it would remove the cancer in its entirety.

Bryan is now on Synthroid, something he will have to take the rest of his life as it mimics the hormones normally produced by thyroid gland. Because the thyroid was removed, chemo wouldn't be necessary.

Bryan grew up in a Christian household and was, as he describes it, a guy who knew how to "play" Christian. I had never heard this term before but believe it describes so many.

He was baptized when he was 12—but says it was to appease dad. Went to a Christian high school. Was a good kid and didn't cause problems, didn't cuss, and was thought to be one of those ideal Christian kids. One problem: he didn't really believe.

On a high school senior trip to North Carolina that included whitewater rafting, bungee jumping, and all the things' kids love there was a Pastor who asked very poignant questions.

The pastor talked about his son, who died at an early age. He then asked all the kids if they knew when their time was coming. He went on to ask: if they didn't, what were they going to do about it?

It was then, May 5, 2000, that Bryan committed his life to Christ and stopped just playing Christian. He got baptized, again, this time because he *wanted* to. It was this faith in God that got him through the move, got him through the time his wife was in the hospital after Jonah was born. And got him through cancer.

Of course, he, like so many others, thought "why me, God?" He then recalled the Bible verses he learned as a kid: *I can do all things through Christ who strengthens me* (Philippians 4:13). Then also *Do all things without murmurings and disputing's: That ye may be blameless and harmless, the sons of God, without rebuke, in the midst of a crooked and perverse nation, among whom ye shine as lights in the world* (Philippians 2:14-15).

Bryan doesn't question God anymore. He realizes that if he and his family hadn't moved, the chances are that his cancer would not have been discovered while it was still treatable.

Case #17:

Jerry-Pancreatic Cancer & a Lesson on Living

I owe so many things in life to Jerry. Over 40 years ago he got me into the franchising business. That necessitated a move to Ohio to work for the franchisor. Six years later I returned to my hometown in Illinois and worked with Jerry for years, eventually becoming a business partner.

He named his business LTM Water after his three kids, Laurie (the oldest), Tom and Mark (who was named after me). Quite an honor.

Jerry was involved with the local Lutheran high school. It was the same Lutheran High where my dad served on the school board when the school opened in the mid-'60s. I videotaped Jerry's basketball games at Lutheran when he was the coach and his son, Tom, was in seventh grade. The team was good. No, great. Jerry knew how to coach young boys and motivate them. As this same team stayed together, they eventually went down state in Tom's junior year and finished fourth in the state of Illinois. I was there.

I remember the night Tom called to tell me he was just named the Lutheran high school basketball coach. Jerry was going to be his assistant. I was so excited for them both.

When Jerry was sixty-five, he was diagnosed with pancreatic cancer. A good friend of both of ours had the same diagnosis and had died just a few weeks before.

Pancreatic cancer is usually fatal, and it was for Jerry. But this isn't a story about how Jerry died. It is about how he lived.

It was July 2012. Jerry just hadn't been feeling well. His back was starting to give him issues and, as much as he hated to go to a doctor, he relented.

His local doctor couldn't find anything. His back was so bad that he wanted to take this to the next level. His first visit was to Mayo Clinic, the Friday before Memorial Day. Their advice? "Stop golfing." Sadly, Jerry really enjoyed golfing. The course was only a mile away and it gave him great relaxation.

Jerry was a classic entrepreneur. I met Jerry when he was a business customer at a finance company where I worked. We drove to a Cleveland suburb to visit the headquarters of a national water treatment business and he was awarded a franchise.

The day Jerry found a location for his business, I was with him. The owner of the building said he could occupy the back half of the building. Days later the owner of the building came in and discovered that Jerry occupied the entire building. Jerry was a "better to ask for forgiveness than permission" type of guy. From then on, his business had the entire building.

Several of his previous sales reps joined him at the new company, including Bill.

About the time of Jerry's back issues, Bill was getting extremely sick. The diagnosis: pancreatic cancer. Bill was not only a close friend, but he was also a 20 year+ employee and had this dreaded disease.

What scared Jerry is that he didn't like pizza anymore. Bill lost his love for pizza shortly before he was diagnosed. As silly as that sounds, that was the first warning sign for Jerry.

Jerry was diagnosed with pancreatic cancer at about 4 p.m. one day in July. By 7:30 there were over seventy-five people at his house. Former players, current players, former employees. Jerry had a message: "I'm going to beat this!"

From the outset the family agreed that he wouldn't receive traditional chemotherapy. They chose to go an alternate route with Vitamin C treatment that was extraordinarily successful in Germany.

He got injections a few times a week. Each treatment took hours. While Jerry was receiving his Vitamin C treatment, he was always selling his company's product. *(No surprise to me!)*

In August, Jerry went into a hospital about fifty miles from his home to see if he could qualify for a new surgical procedure. The Whipple procedure is used to treat tumors and other disorders of the pancreas.

The well-known surgeon from Loyola in Chicago came up to see if he could save Jerry. He told the family that, if he could do it, he would be in the operating room for 8 to 12 hours. If he couldn't, he would be out in 30 minutes.

Mom and the three kids waited anxiously, praying . . . hoping. But the news wasn't good.

In 30 minutes, the surgeon was out. It couldn't be done on Jerry.

When Jerry became too ill to continue running the business, the family members each stepped up to fill his role.

The word about Jerry and his illness spread. One business wanted to hold a fundraiser for him. Jerry and his wife, Barb, had been successful. They told the business they didn't need any money. They would, however, appreciate a fundraiser for a scholarship at Lutheran High School.

Jerry's favorite number was eleven. Throughout his high school and college career playing basketball, football, and baseball, Jerry was #11. Tom and all the grandkids wore #11.

The fundraiser was successful, raising exactly $11,000. Could it be a sign for the family?

Jerry received a card one day that read, "BELIEVE." That would become his and the family's mantra. Prominent at every Lutheran High sporting event during Jerry's illness was a giant banner that read "BELIEVE."

Tom and his dad had been coaching for a couple of years. They took third place in the state before Jerry got sick. It was an outstanding year— especially for a school that didn't have reputation as a basketball powerhouse before Tom and Jerry took over.

Tom shares an event that was truly inspiring:

The team all knew and respected Dad not only as one of their coaches, but also one who has a great basketball mind. It didn't seem like that long ago when he was inducted into his college's Hall of Fame as a player. I was blessed to introduce him that night for his induction.

Dad was too weak to go to the game. He was in the late stages by then. But he had to be there to support his team. We were playing a team that was out to upset us. The first half was back and forth. We walked into the locker room at halftime with a couple point lead.

Dad needed help to make it to the locker room. I can still picture him s l o w l y walking through the room. Each player's eyes riveted on him as he headed toward the bathroom. His face was pale.

It is hard to see a man you've loved your entire life aging by every step of their walk. Yet, he was.

I looked at him, then, looking at the team, I formed a "C" with my left hand. I said to the team, "This is a C. This C stands for COURAGE. That man, your coach, has courage. Courage to leave the house tonight. Courage to be here to support you. Courage to have people help him just so he can come to the locker room. In the next half we'll see how much courage you have – courage to beat a tough foe. Courage to give it your all and move on in the tournament."

We won that game. By twenty-seven points. I've never seen a team more courageous, and more driven, than we were in the second half. Dad had given them the inspiration they needed.

In his last 11 months, Jerry had such an impact on people. Jerry told MK and me how he had baptized a caregiver one day in the hospital. He took every opportunity to witness other patients while receiving his Vitamin C treatments.

He died in May. The 19th to be exact. I know this because it is on my calendar. Has been since he died. Every year I reach out to his kids to let them know I love them and I'm thinking of them that day.

Jerry grew up in a small town about forty miles away from where he and his family lived when he died. The whole family was well known in that small town. When Jerry told his dad they were moving to the "big city," his dad warned him, "Don't do that. No one will know you there and no one will come to your funeral."

I remember the visitation in that "big city." MK and I came up from Texas for it. Over nine hundred people came to the visitation. The line was out the gym of the high school and half-way around the school. We waited 60–90 minutes just to get into the gym. The best part was I was able to talk to so many others I knew, and we'd tell Jerry stories together.

Laurie said they still get phone calls weekly from people asking for their dad. They are regularly approached by people who want to share stories about their dad. One was from a young man at Lutheran. Jerry walked up to him and asked him if he was trying out for the baseball team the next week. The young man said he didn't own a baseball glove and he couldn't.

Jerry told him to get his butt in the car with him, right now, and took him to a sporting goods store and bought him a great glove. That is how Jerry lived. He told his kids, "In order to be a friend, you must make a friend. Listen to people closely." A great lesson for us all.

Case #18:

Dave – Loving Family through Cancer Battles

Family. This story is close to home: it is about one of Mary Kay's relatives. Of course, now my relative. It is a man's perspective about losing one wife to breast cancer, getting married years later, and having his wife, today, also get it.

It is a story about a person who has dealt with cancer his entire life. Mom, dad, and both of his wives.

It is a story about a man's perspective and what a survivor goes through—and continues to go through.

It was the early '90s. Dave was dating Laura. On one of their first dates, he put his hand behind her neck in a show of affection while he was driving and noticed she pulled away. It was then he learned that Laura had had non-Hodgkin's as a senior in college. She didn't want Dave to notice that her hair was much shorter in back than it was on the rest of her head.

Most of all, she was afraid Dave wouldn't date her as he knew she had cancer. Dave was familiar with cancer fear. His mom died of lung cancer in 2000 after a lengthy illness. Later, Dave's dad would get renal cancer. He lived with this, though, for over 20 years, passing in 2012.

At his parents' 40th wedding anniversary, Dave and his siblings decided to have a huge celebration. Privately, they believed that mom wouldn't make it to their 50th. She didn't.

Laura's non-Hodgkin's came back when she and Dave were engaged. She had radiation previously. Then , full chemotherapy results in changing the date of the wedding. The kids were looking at the wedding pictures one day and asked why mom had such full hair at the wedding, but shorter hair on the honeymoon. They didn't realize their mom had worn a wig at the wedding because of the cancer.

When she was cancer-free, they decided to try for kids. Success! Two girls, about five years apart. This was a win for them. Their dreams were coming true, regardless of the earlier health challenges.

In 2006 Laura got breast cancer. The oncologist looked at her file and noticed it was quite thick. After studying it further, the doctor had an aha moment and shared it with them. It was about the radiation Laura had from the non-Hodgkin's. Over 50% of those who had the type of radiation she'd taken developed breast cancer years later.

Laura needed chemotherapy. She had her lifetime limit on radiation.

Dave noticed that people with cancer usually have mood changes. Either they are so happy to be alive—or they are so angry they have cancer.

It seemed to Dave that the worst health news always came when he was traveling for his job. It was September 17, 2015. Dave saw on his cell phone that his daughter, then a senior in high school, had called. He was in the middle of a meeting and let it go to voicemail. Seconds later she called again. Then his mother-in-law called. He excused himself and took the call. Laura was in the hospital once again.

Immediately Dave left and meeting and jumped in a cab to the airport to fly home to the east coast from Chicago O'Hare. While in the cab, he got a call that the doctor needed to talk to him. The next words were "your wife has expired." What a way to find out that the love of your life died.

On the flight home lightning struck his plane. All Dave could think was, *this is great. My kids are going to lose both parents, on the same day, due to two unrelated circumstances!*

Laura's death wasn't planned. They hadn't planned.

The first year was a fog. Work didn't help, so he switched jobs—but took time off first. He went to grief counseling. The counselors told Dave he was doing great. Dave didn't feel that. He drank too much. That didn't help either.

Eventually he met Heather.

Heather's husband had died of brain cancer in 2008. She had two daughters, the eldest the same age as his youngest daughter. The two daughters even knew each other and were friends.

Eventually, Dave and Heather fell in love and planned a wedding.

It was April 10, 2020, the morning of their wedding, when Heather asked him to feel this lump in her breast and asked him what he thought. He knew on his wedding day what that meant.

Heather had stage 3 breast cancer. Their honeymoon period was a series of doctor and oncology visits. She ended up at Sloan-Kettering Cancer Center in New York. COVID was at its peak and Dave couldn't go into any of the appointments with her.

In their first year of marriage Heather went through chemo—then radiation.

I can't imagine the emotions their four girls were going through, especially Dave's two girls. Twice they faced losing someone to cancer.

Today Heather is doing well. She has been cancer-free for two years. The testing and oncologist appointments are ongoing—but she remains cancer-free.

Her faith helps her through the challenges.

Dave knows that radiation and chemo can take a toll on patients. He is impressed with the attitude Heather has. It is great in private and great in public.

I'm reminded that the unrecognized victim of cancer is the caregiver—the wife, the husband, the parent of someone who has cancer. It is a lesson to never forget.

Case #19:

Marlene–Gum Cancer at 85

Picture your mother or your grandmother being diagnosed with gum cancer at age 85. Before I heard this story I simply would have thought, "She has lived a great life! We will make sure that we do all we can to have her feel appreciated and loved as she lives out her remaining days."

In fact, if it is me at 85, unless I'm spry and lively, have all my faculties and am still playing bocce ball and putt putt with great grandkids, this is what I would tell MK and my kids to do.

85?! I don't think I could withstand Marlene's ordeal.

I learned about her story from her son, Rob. Years ago, MK and I hosted Marlene's son and daughter-in-law, Rob, and Alex, in our Florida home along with their six-year-old twins. He was one of the few sales professors in the country at a university that offered a degree in professional sales.

The twins are now college sophomores. Over those 13 years we've remained friends.

January 10, 2022, Marlene fell and broke her left arm and wrist. As Marlene describes it, "I'm right-handed. It wasn't that bad."

Alex and Rob insisted that she rehabilitate at their house. Her meat was cut for her, jars were opened, nothing major, really. Within two weeks she was chomping at the bit to return to her home.

Over the years Marlene has religiously gone to her primary care dentist and her periodontist. Both knew that she had oral lichen planus, a common disease that causes inflammation, for more than 10 years. Her gums were receding.

Marlene used a particular ointment when the symptoms reoccurred. They would come and go, and she was told to reduce any stress in her life to help. Over the years she had two molars on the lower left jaw replaced with implants. She also a skin graft to the gum area of one implant with tissue from the roof of the mouth, as the gums were getting worse. The periodontist recommended another graft from the roof of her mouth because the second implant had gum that was now receding. Diet changes were required to prevent injuring her gums.

A month after breaking her bones, Marlene had the second skin graft surgery. This time the periodontist took tissue and sent it to a laboratory for a biopsy. A week later the stitches were removed. The phone rang and Marlene was surprised to hear the periodontist wanted to see her again. Marlene asked the staff on the phone if she could speak on the phone instead. The answer was "no"! Strange.

A February 15 appointment was set. At the appointment, the periodontist told Marlene that the biopsy revealed cancer of the gums. When she heard the results of the biopsy, she didn't react, she was simply numb.

Marlene was offered a specialist who is skilled at treating her type of cancer, but she wanted to be treated at the closest hospital to her house. One that she knew well and could easily drive to. Her three sons disagreed and told her she really needed to do this at Northwest Memorial Hospital—a well-respected hospital in Chicago. On a good day this was a 45-minute drive. In Chicago snow or heavy Chicago traffic, it is at least double that time.

March 24th was the scheduled five-to-six-hour surgery. Hers took 12 hours. Doctors told her that at her age, without being in incredibly good health, with a strong heart and lungs, she wouldn't have survived it. Multiple surgery teams removed six teeth from the bottom left of her mouth along with a portion of her gums, scraping her jawbone to ensure no cancer cells were left.

She recovered in the hospital, then transferred to a rehab center. Marlene's three sons took two-week shifts spending every day with mom.

A fissure had opened in her mouth that allowed food particles to become trapped and a raging infection ensued. Her face swelled beyond recognition. Back to the hospital for another surgery.

The surgeons assured her they had removed **all** the cancer. The lymph nodes were clear. As a result of this she wouldn't need radiation or chemo.

She couldn't eat, so the hospital inserted a feeding tube to deliver nutrients. At some point the tube stopped working. Back to the hospital for another surgery and anesthesia. The doctors proclaimed that the problem was fixed. They thought she'd be in the hospital another 12 days. No such luck. Again, the feeding tube just fell out, back for another surgery. But "third time's a charm;" the feeding tube was finally secure. The ordeal was mentally and physically exhausting. She experienced hallucinations.

Two months from the initial surgery she got to go home—actually, to her son Rob's home in suburban Chicago. He and his wife, Alex, treated her to what Marlene would say was gourmet meals, albeit without her favorite—steak.

What Marlene feared most was her loss of independence. She didn't want to have to rely on her sons to survive. This motivated her to fully embrace her exercises. She routinely worked eight to ten hours a day on in-home exercises for her arms, legs, back, and speech.

She had been in bed for so long that her muscles had atrophied. She had to build them back slowly. Her favorite exercise was sticking her tongue out at Rob, knowing it was part of her rehab.

After in-home exercises she graduated to more difficult outpatient therapy twice a week. She hit her self-imposed goal of walking one mile.

With all this behind her, she and the boys decided it was time for independent living in a two-bedroom apartment. It would be quite a change from the seven-room house she lived in for over 50 years. Everyone was proud and delighted.

Marlene's religion was not a source of comfort for her. For some reason she couldn't pray. She tried to watch mass each week on TV but just couldn't focus on the 30-minute program. She thinks she was angry with God.

This is slowly changing. She attends a regular Bible study in her community. This is new for her, as she grew up in the Catholic church where the priests read the Bible, not the parishioners. She is enjoying this new chapter in her life.

All she needs now is to replace those teeth. Alex drives Marlene around Chicagoland seeing different professionals who could help the next step in the process.

They don't know for sure if it can all be one with one surgery until they get in there. Marlene will need help again, so it will be back to Rob and Alex's for more rehabilitation. She isn't worried. She knows she will finally get her steak when the new teeth are in place.

Case #20:

Nancy & John – Prostate Cancer that Metastasized.

Nancy and I went to high school together. She was just a year younger than me. We even dated a couple of times in high school.

Don't think I've talked to her for almost 50 years. Her story is one, though, that makes me cry, then makes me cheer, then makes me cry again, and, finally, makes me cheer!

It reinforces the point that we have no idea what anyone is going through at any given time. Just because they are great today doesn't mean they will be fine tomorrow. And vice versa. Nancy's story illustrates this vividly.

N ancy and John had been married for 21 years. He was a jerk. A raging alcoholic. He was so bad that, coming home from Nancy's 40th birthday party, he threw all her presents out of the window of the car, over the guardrail into the ravine. What provoked him to do this was the balloons from her party. They were hitting him on the head as he drove, and this started his nastiness.

Finally, Nancy had had enough. It was time to plan for a divorce. The kids were 10 years apart. Keith was still in high school, Renee in grade school.

Nancy was in the medical profession, teaching new office people how to do billing for the doctors. She had an excellent job with a national company. Besides the issues with John, life was good.

John was a stickler for his lawn and how it looked. He went out to mow on a hot August day. Nancy brought icy water out to him a couple of times, but he was glad to come in the kitchen when he finished for more water. He passed out. Nancy called his best friend, who rushed over to see what he could do. By this time John woke up, claimed he was fine, but complained about his shoulder and how badly it hurt.

A couple of days later, John went to the doctor, who immediately required rotator cuff surgery. After a couple of weeks of healing, John started physical therapy in early October. By November, nothing was helping— he still had the same pain.

The doctor decided to do an MRI of the rotator cuff, then decided to do a scan of his body to see if there was anything else to be concerned about. Nancy said the scan "lit up like a leopard." Spots everywhere.

She knew it meant cancer. John hadn't yet. One specialist sent John to another one—an oncologist.

Nancy knew of the oncologist to whom John was referred. He had an excellent reputation. Once the two men were in his office, John asked him exactly what kind of doctor he was— his specialty. This was the first-time cancer had been mentioned to John. Their first appointment was on December 26th. Nancy remembers the date well.

The X-rays weren't good. His doctor knew he needed a biopsy ASAP. A neurosurgeon was recommended. Then a radiologist. No one wanted to take the case. The largest tumor was at the base of his skull— so large that it would push John's head forward when he stood or walked.

Finally, the neurosurgeon agreed he would do it. He needed to take a tissue sample from the tumor and see what kind of cancer it was. The doctor took three tissues samples—one was sent to Mayo Clinic, another to somewhere in Bethesda, Maryland, and the third remained at his treatment hospital.

The results came back. Bleak: prostate cancer that had metastasized throughout John's body. The prognosis was that he had six months to live.

About this same time the office where Nancy worked was closing. All the records need to go to one of the main offices in downtown Chicago two hours away. Because Nancy was a supervisor, and because records, back then, were all written, she personally brought them to the Chicago office. They needed her to stay and help go through them all, and the company put her up in a charming hotel in downtown Chicago. Corporate management was impressed by her knowledge and quality of her work and offered a position in Chicago. They were so insistent they offered to buy her house and give her a great salary.

Nancy told them, "My husband is dying, my daughter is in grade school, and I don't want to raise her in Chicago. I appreciate it but need to turn you down. My life is about to change, and I have no idea what direction it will take."

Little did she know it would be a blessing—a blessing she believes that was from God.

John insisted that the family take all the trips they never took before, trying to jam everything into the next six months. John and Nancy tried all diverse kinds of natural foods. They even looked for other types of treatment.

The doctor recommended radiation through John's neck. He lost his appetite for food. He lost his appetite for liquor. John's issues with alcohol were gone.

Nancy liked they were finally a real family.

Her brother-in-law, a devout Christian, offered to take John on a fishing trip to Alaska. John came back a new person. No longer an agnostic. Now a committed Christian. He wanted them to find a church and get involved. This same person now did Bible studies at church on Wednesday evenings. Of course, church every Sunday.

Trips everywhere including Disney World with the kids. It was all about family now. He went fishing in Alaska a couple more times. Also, a trip to Puerto Rico. Life was about togetherness.

He always wanted a big deck at the back of his house. They had one built while John supervised. They talked for hours. Talked about stuff they had never talked about before.

John's bones were now brittle. One day while Nancy was out, she reminded John not to try to answer the phone. He did, fell, and broke his arm. Back to the doctor, who put the arm in a sling. The doctor told John it was time to look at hospice.

John woke up Saturday morning to tell Nancy he was ready. She called the doctor and let him know. First, he wanted to confirm with John. They called a hospice center, and within hours the center brought them a hospital bed, wheelchair, commode, and other items he might need.

To make space in their bedroom, Nancy gave away the furniture they had used for 21 years. She had a single bed delivered so that she could sleep next to John's hospital bed.

That first day, the two of them talked all night. When someone is dying, Nancy said, you never run out of things to talk about.

John apologized. Apologized for his drinking. Apologized for how he treated her. Asked her what he could do to make up for those years of misery he gave her. They held hands each night, all night.

Their house was full of visitors and friends. Friends from the church who just wanted to pray with them. People from John's work. Family. People were always there visiting this new man named John.

One night John dropped Nancy's hand. She didn't realize that this was part of the dying process and that he wouldn't be alive much longer.

Hospice came the next morning. They saw the signs. They shaved John. Put his favorite shirt on him. Sprayed cologne on him. About noon they told Nancy to get on the phone and invite people to come over ASAP.

Nancy's sister was staying with her, sleeping on the couch, to help however she could. Nancy called John's best friend and told him to bring any of his friends who would like to see him one last time. Her sister called all the family members who lived close by.

Both told everyone they called, "John is going to pass today."

Nancy played Joyce Meyer messages and songs. In the end, Nancy and John's favorite nieces were with him. He opened his eyes, looked at them, then closed his eyes for the final time.

That evening the house was full of family and friends. Sharing their love for the two of them. Praying. Hugging. Crying.

He had only been in hospice care for one week. But John knew what was coming even though Nancy didn't want to admit it.

If Nancy's job hadn't had left town, she wouldn't have had the severance package, wouldn't have been able to spend three wonderful years with John. Wouldn't have spent the time with mom.

As I've heard before, when God closes a door, He opens a window.

The next summer Nancy and daughter, Renee, spent time with Nancy's brother in Connecticut. It was a wonderful time even before her brother surprised them with a trip to NYC. Her brother had connections as he was an extraordinarily successful newspaper executive. They got tickets for the front row for the Broadway musical, CATS. Still, all these years later, Renee's favorite music.

Nancy's son, Keith, a young man by this time, was in a committed relationship with his girlfriend and opted to stay in town. Nancy and daughter Renee enjoyed a time to build a relationship that wasn't about death and dying. It helped form the relationship they still have today.

After returning home from Connecticut, Nancy considered a new career. As school approached Nancy dropped off a résumé at a local college. It was a Tuesday. The phone was ringing as she walked in the door. She started there the following Monday. God works in mysterious ways!

She still had the church family. She and Renee continued going on Sundays and Wednesday nights. Nancy was also a Girl Scout leader.

Nancy was at this point in her forties. Time passed, and she started thinking it would be nice to have companionship.

The local paper published a personal page with pictures of people who would like companionship. All legitimate. She highlighted a couple of names and contacted a couple of them. One gentleman, Pat, caught her eye as he loved the smell of lilacs. They found a way to contact each other and had a great first phone call. A couple of hours long.

After many phone calls they agreed to meet. He lived less than 20 miles away, kids were grown and had grandkids. She found out he owned his own house, had a 30+ year job, and was the same age as Nancy. Plus, he was deeply religious—he'd grown up in the Catholic church and stayed active there his entire life.

A year later, Nancy and Pat got married. Eighteen years into their marriage, they were walking to a fireworks display when Pat announced he couldn't walk any longer. A doctor diagnosed heart disease and inserted stents in his legs that would give him a couple more years to live. One day while Pat was cutting a pool liner, his knife slipped, and he severely cut his foot. Pat underwent surgery to open the blood flow to his foot so it could heal.

Soon he was healing well and feeling fine, so Nancy joined high-school girlfriends at a cabin a couple of hours away. At the end of the evening, she called Pat and was concerned about how he sounded. She told her friends she would drive back home in the morning.

When she got home Saturday morning, he wasn't fine. Something wasn't good. Pat was perspiring terribly. Keith came over to help Nancy get him in the truck to get him to the hospital.

Soon Nancy found out the wound had been infected, and the infection had made its way to his brain. The doctors scheduled surgery for the next morning. The family was there, and Pat assured them all would be fine.

While he was in surgery, Nancy heard "Code Blue in Surgery" over the PA. She knew. It was Pat.

Pat came out of surgery after the Code Blue. He was in an induced coma until he could go back into surgery. Back in surgery they had to amputate Pat's leg. When Pat was back in his room Nancy noticed that his "good leg" was badly swollen.

Back to surgery the next morning. Pat assured the family that all was well and in God's care.

Pat didn't make it back into surgery the next morning. He died in the ICU just as Nancy was walking back into the hospital to see him that next morning before surgery.

It was September 14. Pat was only sixty-two. He had always urged Nancy to retire at 62. She gave her notice at the career college where she taught that this would be her last semester. It was.

Think about this. You are sixty-two. You have had two husbands die. Like most would do, Nancy asked God, "Why me? What have I done to make you angry?"

In the next couple of months Nancy turned her help to one of her girl-friends from high school. Severe drinking problem. She was one of the girls at the cabin that weekend. Those girls performed an intervention and got her into a hospital. Same hospital where I was born!

Her husband took her out of the hospital. Said she didn't need it. Nancy knew better. She and the other girlfriends helped keep her alive. Kept her positive. Told her that life was worth living.

But a month later she was dead. Drank herself to death.

Was God mad at Nancy? Just the opposite. He knew she was a wonderful caregiver.

The three years with John after his diagnosis were the best three years of their life together. She was there for her mom before she died. She was there with Pat as he went through his heart and surgery issues before he died. And she did her best with her great friend, who desperately needed her help. She helped get her into full-time treatment.

Nancy is a caregiver. Along the journey she now knows that God put her into that role. She learned, at each challenge she had, that He was guiding her how and where she needed to be.

This is one satisfying life story for her.

Laura & Husband, Mike's, Kidney Transplant

Family. When a divorce happens, as it did for me when I was thirty, you don't realize that the "family" you saw each week, shared Thanksgiving and Christmas with and other fun events, might not be in the picture much longer after the divorce. But I stayed in touch with that side of the family as my kids are still close to them.

I stay connected with several of them thanks to Facebook, but there are others who I haven't talked to in almost 40 years.

We lived close to Aunt Betty Ann, Uncle Jake, and their kids, Michael, Laura, James, and Paul, when we lived in Rockford. But once we moved away, I lost track of their lives. Laura was the second of their four. I can easily pick her out in her second-grade picture, but doubt if I would pick her out of a dozen people in a crowd today.

Uncle Jake passed away in 2020 at the age of eighty-six with numerous health issues (bladder cancer, diabetes, and Parkinson's disease). Aunt Betty Ann is still alive today. What Laura has endured is an amazing story. Her story is quite different.

I t had been a struggle for Laura and Mike. Their first child, Sam, was stillborn. Being raised Catholic, Laura thought her priest would have answers to help her. She never received the answers she hoped for. Their second son, Ethan, was born prematurely at 32 weeks and had an extended stay in the NICU followed by years of health complications. Their third son, Lucas, was born with complications.

When Laura's husband, Mike, was sixteen, he found out he had polycystic kidney disease (PKD).

According to the Mayo Clinic, PKD is an inherited disorder in which clusters of cysts develop primarily within the kidneys, causing the kidneys to enlarge and lose function over time. Cysts are noncancerous round sacs containing fluid. The cysts vary in size, and they can grow exceptionally large. Having multiple cysts or large cysts can damage the kidneys.

Mike's grandfather had had it. His dad had it. One of two of his dad's sisters had it, and three of her children died from it. Both of Mike and Laura's sons have the disease. Older son, Ethan, now has just 52% kidney function at age 25.

This also means that Mike can never get life insurance. Neither can Ethan and Lucas.

Mike and his son, Ethan, were wrestling in the backyard when Mike fell. Both kidneys bled and clots formed, causing blockages. Once that happened, it was time to consider a transplant.

Mike had been treated locally for the condition for years and was informed he had to wait until he only had 15% kidney function to get on the transplant list. Due to care issues at the local hospital following his kidney injury, Laura had him transferred to a well-known hospital within a couple of hours of their home. The University of Wisconsin's hospital in Madison had a great reputation.

It was a great decision. They told them that at 30% kidney function, he could start the process to get on the transplant list, though he ordinarily wouldn't begin accruing time until his kidney function was at 15%. But with an incurable condition like his, there was the chance to accrue time earlier.

It looked like it would be less than a year before there would be a cadaver donor. But then changes to UNOS (United Network for Organ Sharing) allocation rules caused Mike's wait time to change from less than one year to almost four.

While Mike was accruing time on the list for a cadaver donor, he and Laura were also searching for a living donor, as outcomes from living donors are much better than those from cadavers. Laura was shocked to see the number of people who raised their hand, across the country, to help. One of those people was a person Laura worked with, Lisa.

Laura and Lisa didn't know each other, as Lisa was a remote agent. However, their manager suggested they might want to connect as Lisa had just gone through the kidney transplant process with her husband, Rick. The four met one day over breakfast, Lisa decided she wanted to be tested to be a donor. Lisa's husband, Rick, had received a live donor from his brother-in-law, and, seeing how life-changing it was for her husband, Lisa wanted to pay it forward.

While others went through the testing process, Lisa discovered she was a match for Mike. However, she was over the weight threshold for donation, and she would have to lose those extra pounds before she could donate.

She spent the next year on a strict regime of exercising and eating correctly with a goal of becoming Mike's donor. Eventually she lost one hundred pounds. Lisa describes it as that she and Mike saved each other's lives. Mike got her kidney, and she changed every facet of her life. Today she works out, eats right, and has maintained a healthy weight!

Lisa never mentioned these challenges and her weight loss to anyone she worked with. She worked out of her house and coworkers had no idea. Laura worked in an office, though, and loved to tell the story of what Lisa did for her family.

When Mike went into surgery, the two boys were only 16 and 11.

Both of Mike's kidneys were so enlarged that the surgeons had to perform a bilateral nephrectomy, removing both kidneys during the surgery. Scar tissue had formed through the years and his kidneys were adhered to his intestines, diaphragm, and pancreas, which led to serious complications after exercising them.

Laura remembers driving up to Madison and calling her brother, James, who was a paramedic. James helped her understand that she had to be the strong one for the family now and to tackle the problem in front of her and not look beyond that. That is what she did, one obstacle at a time. Most importantly, she needed to be there for Mike.

Since then, Laura has received a lesson in dealing with medical establishments. And it hasn't been a pleasant experience—especially after COVID.

Mike was exposed to COVID-19. He tested negative at the time but started having depression and anxiety issues. Upon seeking admission to a psychiatric facility with suicidal ideations, Mike tested positive for COVID. It was later theorized that he had contracted COVID-19 upon his return to work and the psychiatric issues he experienced were part of COVID psychosis.

Mike had long COVID. He developed a myriad of complications: physical, psychological, and neurological. He is currently being treated by a long-COVID clinic at Northwestern in Chicago, a memory care clinic, and an epilepsy neurologist at UW Health University Hospital in Madison, WI. Dizziness and seizures post-COVID led to a fall that caused a complete rotator cuff tear, leaving him unable to use his left arm for much of anything. Unfortunately, due to his neurological issues, he is not a candidate for a shoulder replacement because he poses a fall risk.

He was, and still is, denied disability. He hasn't been able to work for the past two years since his COVID diagnosis, due to the long COVID and his complicated medical situation.

I asked Laura if she'd ever gotten mad at God. She hasn't. She grew up in a world, however, that instructed people if they were good people and did the right things, they would never have anything bad happen to them.

She has learned this isn't true.

She values having good doctors, and having cousins she can reach out to for help—one a retired nurse.

Case #22:

Carol-Sinus Abscess to the Brain

Not all harrowing stories are about life-threatening issues. Some concern life-altering issues that leave scars lasting 50 years. Those scars can be physical as well as emotional. Such is this story about Carol.

It was the 1970s when Carol suffered what started as a simple sinus infection. Simple is the wrong word. Carol's face was swollen, eyes were swollen shut, and she had an extreme sensitivity to light. She wasn't aware of behavior changes, but people at work commented that she seemed angry all the time and had bad mood swings. How bad? She told her boss to get bent (not in those exact words—hers were a bit more colorful).

Back then one didn't need to see a doctor for simple ailments. Normal antibiotics took care of things. But a week of taking antibiotics didn't help, so she went in to get her sinuses drained. This would cure it, she thought.

A couple more weeks brought on another sinus infection. Back to the doctor, who shined a light on Carol's eyes and saw that her eyes didn't dilate. This wasn't a sinus infection—something much worse. The doctor told her to get to the hospital—NOW. The rest is a haze.

She threw up and passed out in the elevator leaving the doctor's office. The next thing she remembers is that she was in the hospital. Her ex-husband had taken her there. The doctor she first saw asked her a series of easy questions: names of kids, years they were born, and so forth. But she couldn't answer anything the doctor quizzed her on.

The next day, however, she felt fine. Took a shower and thought she was ready to go home. But the nurses had more tests for her. After the tests, they

101

brought her back to a different room—one in the ICU. Carol was more confused than ever. Carol remembers:

> *A nurse comes and announces she is going to shave my head. I say, "Excuse me, you are going to do what!" She tells me again she is going to shave my head. My response is "you and whose army!" Well, she left the room and came back with the army. My head is now completely shaved. My hair at that time was down to the middle of my back. This nurse comes back in with a paper bag. I ask what is in the bag and she tells me it is my hair. I ask her what I am supposed to do with it, glue it back on? She tells me by state law they must give it to me. I promptly threw the hair in the bag into the hall and told her that is what I think about the law. Of course, it goes everywhere in the hall.*

She was getting medicines through an IV. A week later she woke up, still in the ICU. She had been in a drug-induced coma for a week. She didn't realize that she had gone through eight hours of brain surgery. Looking in the mirror, she saw two black eyes, bandages on her head, and a swollen face. Still with no idea why she had brain surgery, she spent another week in ICU. Going to the bathroom required a nurse holding her up on each side so she wouldn't fall – even when her mother and sister were there, as well as other visitors.

The pain was so intense at times during the night (what felt like burning in the veins) that she pulled out the IV in her sleep. More tests. More medicine. Finally, a regular room with a parade of medical specialists including infectious disease doctors, students, internal medicine physicians, neurologists, and, finally, the doctor who had done the operation.

Finally, she understood why all of this was happening. At first, the doctor thought she had a brain tumor and that it was important to operate immediately. To determine if it was cancerous, they had to remove part of her skull. Her family was told she may never speak or walk again and had no guarantee what "normal" functions she would have.

Surgery revealed it wasn't a tumor. It was an abscess. The pus in the sinus infection had broken through the sinus membrane and caused the abscess. Quickly, the infection had spread to Carol's brain.

Carol became a case for the School of Medicine. She remained in the hospital for a full month and, today, has soft spots in her head, like those of a newborn. She still has a scar across her scalp from ear to ear. Fortunately, her thick hair covers the scar well.

After the surgery Carol suffered grand mal epileptic seizures. Carol had no warning signs when they would occur. One time she was driving her full-sized conversion van with her mother in the car when she had a seizure and took out nine mailboxes, went airborne, and slammed into a utility pole, snapping it off the ground. Live wires were on the ground. They were in a tight spot financially at the time: she and her husband had work hours cut and had decided to let their car insurance go so they could keep their home and keep food on the table. The van was totaled.

She lost her driver's license for five years and had to pay to replace the utility pole.

Eventually, she found the right doctor, who prescribed a cocktail of medications that have allowed her to live without seizures for the past 25 years.

Through all her hardships, Carol looks back and knows that God and His angels were looking out for her. She thanks God every day in her daily prayers.

In Carol's case, being seizure-free has been a blessing. Her memories are still fresh. She concluded with this:

> *Although it wasn't a life-threatening situation, it was a life-altering situation. It was also a scary time not knowing what was happening. Every experience in life, good or bad, makes you a stronger, better person. God envisioned a plan for me since the beginning of time. I strive to live that plan every day. No matter what that plan is, He is never wrong! I just ask*

Him every day to lead me, challenge me, and guide me. Walk with me along the path to fulfill the plan best I can and help me become a better person.

Case #23:

Mary - Leukemia then a Double Mastectomy

I have known Mary for so long I remember calling her "Mrs. H." We went to the same church when I was in eighth grade. Her sons went to the same grade school as I did. Mary started a preschool there—Little Lambs—that is still in operation today. Her husband, Maury, died of non-Hodgkin's lymphoma five years ago. When I was fifteen, only 53 years ago, Maury would pick me up every Tuesday night so I could bowl on his church team in a league.

Yes, we go back. I remember that Maury was in the service and had a Navy tattoo on his upper arm. Maury told his five boys that this is one of those stupid things kids do when they are young, and they should not do the same.

When the boys were young men, they decided to give their dad a special memory for Christmas. They all got duplicate tattoos on their arms, matching dad's—what a great surprise!

Delightful story. Great family. I'm so glad I had a chance to know this family and reconnect with Mary at this stage of her life.

In 2007 Mary went to her primary care physician feeling tired. They did lab work, and everything looked fine. She came back some time later and told her doctor that she would still feel worn out. The doctor took her labs again and admitted to Mary that the last lab was smudged, whatever that meant.

She had a slow-moving type of cancer—chronic lymphocytic leukemia.

With time on her hands Mary enjoyed reading. Ironically, she read a story in Prevention magazine about brain cancer. Her goal was to try and keep the white blood cells and the red cells in a "normal" range—even though she had cancer. If she could do this, she could avoid chemo as well as radiation.

Mary concentrated on eating healthy, avoiding processed foods. She ate antioxidants, such as fruits, vegetables, nuts, seeds, pomegranate juice, and green tea. Her white count was too high, so she decided to tweak her diet a little more and start reading the ingredients for every packaged food she purchased. Mary avoided foods with chemicals and preservatives, and each time she went to the doctor, the white count was lower. It took five years to get the white count to the normal range, but both white and red have been in the normal range ever since she got them there!

The result: she never needed chemo or radiation.

Mary read an article that said people with her type of leukemia used lived only 15 more years. Years later another article changed this length of life to 5-10 years. Again, it has been 16 years for Mary.

Nine years ago, she was diagnosed with breast cancer. She remembered that her sister-in-law had had breast cancer and had a mastectomy. Not long later, she developed breast cancer in the other breast.

Mary decided to have a mastectomy of both breasts simultaneously.

She took an estrogen blocker and was able to avoid chemo or radiation once again! Another blessing from God.

Mary later developed squamous cell carcinoma on her face. It was removed without any other cancer complications.

Last May, Mary—now 85—had a tightness in her chest that doctor's thought might be heart problems. The tightness was, and still is, in her upper abdomen. She went to a gastroenterologist.

The doctor couldn't figure out what it was so decided she would start with an endoscopy. They were both surprised when it showed a tumor—especially in the past three months before she had a PET scan which showed no cancer except for the leukemia, which she still had from 15 years before (but was in check).

She was diagnosed with GE junction cancer.

Gastric cancer starts in the stomach or in the gastroesophageal (GE) junction. The GE junction is where the esophagus (the tube that carries food from the throat to the stomach) meets the stomach.

Stomach cancers tend to develop slowly. Pre-cancerous changes often occur in the inner lining (mucosa) of the stomach.

The doctor detailed options for treatment.

The right way of curing this was extensive surgery that would remove a substantial portion of the esophagus. Part of stomach as well. The upper part of the esophagus is then connected to the remaining part of the stomach. Part of the stomach, then, is pulled up to the chest to become the new esophagus.

Mary chose not to have the surgery.

Instead, she started light chemo but found she just could not manage it. So, she opted not to take it at all.

That was May of 2022. She was given 3–9 months to live. As of January 2023, seven months later, she was doing ok. Today she is fatigued.

Recently she decided to meet one of her sons for pizza after he got off work. It was the first time she'd been out of the house in quite a while. She took four doses of Imodium before leaving the house. Still, she suffered diarrhea. Mary decided it was much easier to have family over to the house as she had at Christmas. And God willing, she plans to do that for Easter.

Mary has, and has always had, an amazing faith. She knows that she has lived longer than most people. She has four wonderful sons (one died years ago), nine grandchildren, and eight great-grandchildren.

The tumor has not grown. If it does, it will cut off her ability to swallow.

Mary does not look at her situation as the end of life. She knows when her earthly life is over it will be the beginning of a new life in Heaven. She will be with Maury again. The picture of Mary's future is bright.

What a wonderful lesson for us all!

Case #24:

Christina - Lymphoma

Christina's is a story about having non-Hodgkin's lymphoma.
Twice. It is a story about survival, patience, friends, and prayer.
It is a story about being told that what you have is inoperable.
You are terminal. You will die.
We were introduced by a good friend of 10 years who was one
of our Glass Doctor franchisees. Thank you, Marilyn!

It was Monday, October 4, 2014. Christina and her husband had just returned to southwest Florida after visiting family up north in Ohio. She noticed that her ears still felt plugged up but assumed this was from the flight home. But then Christina began blacking out and acting strangely.

She regularly lost track of time and fell asleep all the time, even while at work or while driving. Once, she woke up in her garage with the engine running—and had no idea how she got there.

People reported seeing all sorts of crazy stuff on her Facebook posts. One crazy post stated she had not eaten for days. Her husband posted a picture showing everyone, while she was writing this, that he was indeed giving her food.

Christina and her husband were big Ohio State Buckeyes fans. One game day, they had a houseful of people over to watch the football game. People at the party noticed Christina's odd behavior. They contacted her nurse practitioner friend, who told Christina's husband that he should take her to a hospital or doctor to see what was going on.

But Christina knew—it was just an ear infection! Even while in the emergency room, she was doing crazy Facebook posts. Her husband was inundated with phone calls, asking what was going on because her posts weren't making sense.

She went to the hospital on a Saturday in October 2014, and woke up the following Tuesday—with no memory of what had happened. She did notice, though, that there was something sticking out of her skull: a tube that fed fluid into a jar. She had fluid in the brain, which was what was causing the blackouts and memory loss. The doctor asked if she remembered talking to him in the ER, but she didn't. He then told her, not so gently, that the tests showed she had a brain tumor.

Gut punch.

Then he told her the shocking news: it was cancer. Non-Hodgkin's lymphoma can form tumors throughout the body. Her tumor was in a part of her brain that made it inoperable. She was labeled terminal. Another gut punch. Needing time to process this and wanting to know her options, she asked what would happen if she did nothing right away. The doctor told her this cancer would kill her quickly.

The doctor in the local hospital in southwest Florida wanted to start with radiation. Chris had to make a quick decision, which was not easy for her. She was scared. Her mother died of lung cancer. Her mom survived the first time she had it and had a long remission. But the cancer came back. Lung cancer again. Yes, Mom had been a heavy smoker from an early age. Before this cancer could even be treated, it killed her in 2004.

After three radiation treatments at the local hospital, Chris's tumor shrank by 50%. Great news! The doctor, however, also wanted to do traditional chemo. After two treatments with methotrexate, Chris was in remission. To make sure she stayed in remission, the doctor told her they needed to continue these treatments, which she did until early spring 2015.

Each treatment required a hospital stay that usually lasted five days, sometimes longer. Each time she had a treatment, a "rescue drug" (leucovorin) was administered that pulled the chemo out of her system. She could go home when the methotrexate levels were deemed safe. Then, after a week's rest, she went back to the hospital for more chemo. Chris was very outspoken regarding her care. At one point, she knew she had to take a break, and did so over the Christmas holidays.

She then resumed her course of treatment until March 2015. It looked as if she was cured! Only monthly check ups and blood work. But no such luck.

In December, the cancer was back. She and her oncologist decided to go directly to the Moffitt Cancer Center this time as treatment at the local hospital was not an option. This wasn't convenient. Moffitt is two hours from where Christina lives.

Chris had to have her husband, or a friend drive her to Tampa and back weekly. In the early visits to Moffitt, she would have a friend along who would take notes regarding options. As the patient, you don't always hear everything that is said, so it was helpful to have another set of ears to fill in the blanks.

Her Moffitt doctor was the oncology chair, a friend of her local oncologist. He went into detail about the options available. One was that a port be inserted into her head, allowing them to inject chemo directly into her brain, as near as they could get to the tumor.

They started the chemo injections immediately, which was a weekly treatment and not available at the local hospital, so there was weekly travel to Tampa.

Christina didn't know anything about the second option, stem cell replacement, but learned it was a brutal process. She chose that route as it gave her the best chance to live (a 50/50 chance to make it five years). These treatments would be much more intense. This was a big commitment as she would need to take a battery of tests (physical, mental, blood, spinal tap, and bone marrow) lasting five days at Moffitt, and she also had to get local clearance from her dentist and eye doctor before the stem cell process could be considered. This procedure required her to be in the Moffitt hospital 30 to 45 days—without leaving. Christina was lucky that she was able to use her own stem cells, reducing the requirement to be on anti-rejection drugs.

During this entire journey, Christina would get mentally down at times and at one point was ready to give up. In times like this, a lifelong friend, Debbie , would (in Chris's words) give her a kick in the butt! So would

Marilyn and other close friends. It was Debbie who came to stay ahead of her month-plus admission to Moffitt—and even drove her there to make sure she went in.

On the last day, after all the evaluations had been completed and she was approved, Chris had her stem cells collected. They needed a minimum of two million stem cells. She had a bi-valve port installed and was hooked up to a machine that cycled her blood for eight hours at a time. After those eight hours she went back to the hotel and waited for the phone call advising them whether they'd collected enough, or she'd have to do it again the next day.

Being a firm believer in the power of the mind, Christina got it done in one shot. She had to line up volunteers willing to stay with her after the stem cell transplant until her neutrophils and white blood cell counts were in the safe limit for her to be released. Lucky for her, she had two friends who were able and willing to come help her through the aftercare.

When everything was in order, Christina entered the stem cell ward. She remembers how intimidating this was. The doors are locked behind when the patient enters. This is a sterile environment. Everyone in there is in distinct phases of preparation, completely depleting their immune system.

By this time, her two million stem cells had been cleaned and were stored while she was prepped.

Day one was chemo #1. It was nasty and Chris lost her hair right away. One of the things about Moffitt is how they go the extra mile. There is someone on staff who will shave your head. Someone to go on a walk with you. Someone to come to your room and give you a "healing massage."

Day two was more chemo—nastier than the day before. Each of the three treatments is worse than the previous. Day two was the day she finally had to "lose her cookies." Day three was absolutely the strongest and worst. By this time, you have nothing left of your immune system. No neutrophils. And no hair.

Day five finally arrived: the day you get your "cleaned" stem cells reintroduced to your body. The staff comes in singing "Happy Birthday!" as they are creating a whole new you with a new immune system. Chris now celebrates this day every year as her second birthday.

Christina had to remain in the hospital until her blood work showed that her neutrophils and white blood cells were responding. She still needed weeks of daily follow up, but in Tampa, not in southwest Florida.

During the time she was getting her chemo and stem cells, her friends underwent training in her aftercare. What to watch for, temperature checks, and how to keep their room "Moffitt clean." There are local hotels nearby that contract with Moffitt to maintain an elevated level of cleanliness for these patients.

She remembers that her stem cells were returned on October 24, 2016. And she remembers still being up in Tampa on election night 2016, watching the returns in her room.

But soon, she was finally able to go home.

Christina is a firm believer in mind over matter, the power of prayer, and not being afraid to advocate for yourself. You know you better than anyone else. She felt the power of her prayer warriors and credits to good friends and family that helped keep her spirits up.

All this made it possible to achieve her positive outcome. To this day, her local oncologist calls her his "miracle patient."

Over six years later she feels great. When she reached five years and beat the odds, she hosted a huge party to honor all those that were instrumental in her success.

Her follow up now consists of yearly MRIs and blood work and she hopes to be 'released' this year. She still has the port in her chest, but says it's been her safety net, believing superstitiously that if she keeps it, the cancer won't return. However, she now feels ready to have it removed and end this chapter of her life.

They tell her she is cured of this cancer. It **won't** come back. This doesn't mean she won't get other types of cancer—just not the one she has already beaten twice.

When I asked her how she got through it all, she pointed to three areas: her husband, her close friends, and prayer.

At first, she was mad at God and asked, "why did you do this to me?" She learned to pray her way through those thoughts. Christina's not as independent as she used to be and realizes she wouldn't have been able to get through her stem cell replacement process without help—lots of help. Her relationship with God is stronger. She is grateful for each day and for the people in her life. She sees people through different eyes. She has learned not to judge since you don't know what a person has been through or is going through.

Case #25:

Mom Shares Mikey's Story – Leukemia at 15

As I started authoring this book, I never imagined I would hear a story like this one. In June of 2017 Mikey was 15 years old. The great news is that he is still alive.

The following are excerpts from Facebook posts written by his mom. Keep in mind what it must be like for his parents. I know what we went through for only 40 days until we found that I was cancer-free.

I chose to show more of Mikey's mom's posts in the first few months to give you an idea of what they had to deal with when they got the news. These posts continued for the past five years, – but as time went on, the pace slowed to quarterly or semiannual updates.

That doesn't mean mom had less involvement. It only means what you read in the first six months continued for five years. Yes, five years. I posted enough to give you a full taste of what they went through as parents, the amount of time commitment there was, and what it was like for a 15-year-old kid.

I never had to deal with anything like this. Jae had asthma; Marcus broke his arm when skiing. Andy went into convulsions a couple times as a kid. But nothing like what Mikey's mom has been going through for the past five years.

Image one of your kids or grandkids in their teens. Hint: grab tissues. Try and put yourself into Mikey's mother's shoes: she'd never heard of any of these drugs. She never imagined this would be a concern in their own home.

I'll start with a December 2017 post from Mikey's mom. It gives you a much better picture of who Mike is.
Mikey's mother, the author of the Facebook posts that comprise this story, invites you to join Mikey's group on Facebook. You can find the group by searching #TeamMikey.

December 2, 2017

Some of you know us personally but I don't think we've ever really shared Mikey's story with the rest of our #TeamMikey supporters.

Michael is a 15-year-old high school sophomore. He is the youngest of four (two sisters & one brother) and has a niece and a nephew.

Mikey had been very athletic, playing both football and baseball since he was about seven. You can throw a bit of basketball in there too. He's always been an active kid. He's been playing select baseball year-round for the last several years. He really enjoyed playing ball in school last year and was excited for this year.

Unfortunately, everything came to a halt on June 25, 2017, when he was diagnosed with acute lymphoblastic leukemia (ALL).

Mikey complained that morning of pain up his right side, from under his ribs all the way up to his neck. He hadn't slept the night before because he couldn't breathe without pain. Thinking he must have hurt himself rough housing with his friends at the lake the day before, we immediately went to the nearest urgent care.

When the doc examined him, he saw that his pain was coming from an enlarged spleen and told us that we needed to go to the ER for a CT scan.

The CT scan confirmed a very enlarged spleen. Blood work came back "a little off when evaluated on their new equipment" so the ER doc sent the blood to a lab off-location to confirm.

While waiting for those results, the doc explained that he was sure that Mikey had mono considering reported symptoms like the recent sore throat, swollen lymph nodes, fatigue, and achiness— and then add in the swollen spleen. He gave Mikey a dose of steroids while we waited. Then the lab results came back.

Mikey's white blood count (WBC count) was over 212,000 (a normal count is somewhere between 6,000-10,000). He explained that there was a possibility that Mikey may have something more serious than mono, as his WBC was exceedingly high.

The doctor mentioned that Mikey's symptoms are also known symptoms of leukemia or lymphoma, and he was sending us to one of the children's hospitals for further testing.

I didn't panic at this point; my mind was stuck on mono. I could hear in Mikey's voice that he was upset and scared.

I chose a well-known hospital 45 minutes away because we had just spent our entire Sunday in the ER and this hospital was much closer than driving to the well-known children's hospital ninety miles away. Of course, it helped that I had also heard lots of good things about their hospital.

The hospital we chose sent their people to transport Mikey to Temple. I figured this was precautionary due to the enlarged spleen that could rupture. It felt like an eternity waiting for them to get to the ER for him.

I followed the ambulance down I-35 South, yelling at the traffic and feeling anxious while all I could think about while driving by myself, were the words *leukemia* and *lymphoma*. Yet at the same time, repeatedly reminding myself how utterly absurd those words sounded. *Mono, it's just mono and we'll be home tomorrow,* I said aloud several times on my way to Temple.

This boy is one of the most active kids I've ever known. He had just been out fishing and swimming and rough housing with his friends a few days before diagnosis. He had just finished playing spring ball two weeks prior. Yes, he had recently been complaining about being tired & that his legs were hurting him, but that hadn't stopped him from hanging out with his friends. I figured he needed some more sleep (it was summer , and he stays up all night sometimes) and needed to rest his legs from playing so much ball.

We weren't at the hospital long at all when I walked into his room on the fifth floor and was greeted by the resident doctor. She introduced herself (although I forgot her name once the next part of the conversation took place) and asked us if we knew why we were there. I mentioned a couple of his symptoms, Mono, blah blah blah and that we were sent to McLane Hospital in Temple from the ER for more tests. Her next words were "He has leukemia."

Our entire world stopped in that very moment.

The next several days were a whirlwind with people coming to introduce themselves and a plethora of information, most of which we didn't understand. Thank goodness everyone was OK with the same questions repeatedly.

That sums up the beginning of our new normal.

Since his diagnosis I've done a lot of reading up on ALL and the treatment. The drugs used for chemotherapy are no joke, y'all. They're poison. Period. They all have so many dangerous side effects and, you're deliberately hurting your child now in the hopes of killing the cancer for good.

I've read a lot about childhood cancer these last 5 months. I never knew how common childhood cancer is. I never knew there were so many types of childhood cancers, so many types of leukemia. So many children are diagnosed with cancer every day. Too many!

June 27, 2017

Sunday: Mikey was having pain on the left side up to shoulder. He went to the hospital and was sent to another location for CT and blood work.

They found he had enlarged liver and spleen with high white blood count. They transferred him to another hospital.

Monday: He was diagnosed with Leukemia. There will be tests done to determine which type of leukemia he has, and a treatment regimen will begin.

Today: He had port placed and they did a marrow aspiration and spinal tap. His white blood count is down to normal, but platelets are extremely low, so he got a platelet transfusion. If there are no complications, chemotherapy regimen will begin tomorrow. The surgery went good and he's awake and doing well.

His Diagnosis: T-cell acute lymphocytic leukemia. They say the prognosis is a good one and treatment lasts a total of two years, eight months.

June 28, 2017

The first chemo started around 2:45 and lasted about an hour. The plan is once a week. They gave him anti-nausea meds before, which should last about 12 hours. Praying for minimal nausea.

Also, several have asked what "stage" he is. With leukemia there are no stages. Leukemia is just leukemia. They will, however, know from a bone marrow test how advanced it is, and those results take a few weeks.

The doctor has advised that he can have visitors now but only two at a time. Please continue prayers.

June 30, 2017

The doctors say Mikey is doing great so far. Better than they expected, "White blood cell count has decreased beautifully." Next round of chemo will be tomorrow.

If he continues to do well and we all feel comfortable, he will be able to go home as early as Sunday. Thank you all for your continued thoughts and prayers!

July 1, 2017

He had his second round of chemo today. This medication is known to have more serious side effects than the medications in the first round. He was hopefully coming home tomorrow but we found out today that he has the blood clotting gene that his mom and one of his sisters have, which complicates his treatment some.

Today's chemo med is known to cause clots, so now they're adding blood thinner injections twice a day.

Please keep praying for Mikey and his treatments!

July 2, 2017

Mikey is handling the Lovenox injections well, although he definitely hates them! As of now, it looks like he will be discharged tomorrow afternoon. He is anxious to get home. We had a few obstacles when it came to getting his home prescriptions filled.

The hospital pharmacy isn't contracted with our insurance, HEB initially didn't have one of the medications, and his injections must be filled by a specialty pharmacy and mailed. Tuesday being a holiday caused an issue with receiving it on time and almost prevented his being discharged tomorrow.

We were able to locate four doses at an HEB and we'll have to pay cash price for them. Not important. We will be back in Temple Wednesday morning for round three of chemo and his spinal. Please continue to share our fundraisers and continue to pray. Thank you all.

July 19, 2017

Mikey gets his last chemo of phase 1 today at 10:30. One step closer to winning this battle against leukemia! He's been a champion through phase 1... On to phase 2! Keep fighting, Mikey.

July 22, 2017

Mikey had his last chemo of Induction (phase 1) on Wednesday. He will have a spinal tap and bone marrow aspiration this Wednesday coming up and will begin Consolidation (phase 2) the following week. Consolidation lasts 8-10 weeks. There will (hopefully) be less trips to Temple than we had during Induction, but at least every Wednesday for chemo. Oral chemo will be given at home daily as well. He will be done taking the Dexamethasone Tuesday.

He is anxious for his face to get back to normal! I am anxious for some other things to go back to normal.

His numbers are okay now, so he was able to go to the movies the other day with his uncle and cousins.

August 1, 2017

It will be a long day in Temple today. Mikey's bone marrow results show that his Minimal Residual Disease is 0.00, which is better than the required MRD of 0.01! That's an 80-85% chance or better of being cured! So, Consolidation is starting today!

The first two-hour round of fluids is running now while we wait on lab results to determine if he will need FFP (plasma infusion).

He'll have his umbar puncture in a couple of hours (which he is quite annoyed about, since he is "starving" & can't eat after midnight before the procedure), followed by chemo and finished with two more hours of fluids.

Doc says his appetite may take a nosedive today.

August 2, 2017

For the first time since treatment began, Mikey didn't need plasma yesterday. That means that he doesn't have to be back in Temple again this week. Next appointment will be all day Tuesday for another LP and chemo.

He is now taking an oral chemo at home daily as well as an injection today, tomorrow, and Friday. Not something I am thrilled about having to do.

He was happy to get to Texas Roadhouse last night for dinner. I wondered if he would feel up to it after such a long day in clinic and having an LP and the new chemo medications. He was tired and his back was sore from the LP, but he was determined that was what was going to be for dinner.

Today his back felt a little better. He even went outside this evening to shoot a few baskets with the boys! That's the first time he's gone outside to hang out since his diagnosis!

Made my heart happy.

August 8, 2017

Mikey only had a small dose of meds today at the clinic. We had an 8 a.m. appointment and were done by nine. His labs show that he is anemic, which is expected by the docs. His hemoglobin and RBC have all dropped since last Tuesday.

This explains his recent fatigue and headaches. He must be back Friday morning for RBC infusion. His WBC has also dropped significantly, so we are back to wearing masks if he goes anywhere and being precise and strict about visitors.

He's lost a few pounds since stopping the steroids two weeks ago. I can already see a difference in his face. And his appetite is more normal too.

After clinic, we went next door to the hospital for his LP (which was scheduled for 11:30) hoping we could get in sooner, but that wasn't possible, so we took a little nap while we waited for 11:30. His LP went well, recovery was entertaining as usual.

This kid is funny on the norm, y'all should hear him coming out of anesthesia!

I'm still waiting at Texas Roadhouse to do whatever they need to do about the dinner to donate last week. I'm assuming they will get a check from us here soon. Thank you all again for coming out.

Thank you to everyone who continues to follow our page and Mikey's fight. Thank you all for continuing to keep us in your thoughts and prayers.

August 12, 2017

We spent our Saturday in the ER at McLane's today. Mikey has had a headache for 11 days now, initially thought to have been caused by his anemia. Doc thought he would feel much better after Tylenol and yesterday's infusion.

Unfortunately, he was experiencing significant pain in the back of his head again last night. Seems it hurts the most when he is moving around, sitting up, or standing. We tried laying down a heating pad on the back of his neck/head, I even tried rubbing the back of his neck and head. He eventually fell asleep and slept all night.

I paged the on-call doc this morning, hoping they might call in a prescription for something stronger than Tylenol, but they decided it was best to come in for an MRI to rule out blood clots. (He has a genetic clotting disorder that puts him at a higher risk for clots than the average person.)

The MRI came back perfect.

Thankfully, no clots!

They determined that the headache is a spinal headache caused by the LP. Sometimes the hole in the needle doesn't close right and spinal fluid will leak causing a terrible headache that worsens with movement. They gave him some good stuff via IV and some IV fluids and sent us home. He's been asleep for the past 3 hours.

We will continue fluids, caffeine, and Tylenol as needed and follow up with the doc at Tuesday's appointment.

August 19, 2017

Aside from occasional mild headaches, Mikey has been feeling OK this week. We went to Temple yesterday to have labs run, assuming he would need some sort of blood product as usual, but he didn't. His RBC and hemoglobin were low, but not low enough to have to have an infusion. However, Monday will be a different story.

Tuesday will be week #4 of chemo and LP in this Consolidation phase. He will have a week or two "break" from chemo so that his body can build up more cells, while we will still go in to check his labs and get any needed infusion. Then he will start the second four-week round of chemo to finish Consolidation.

I am profoundly grateful that he has done so well, and all while feeling OK.

I know he is going stir crazy being in the house constantly. But dad will be home today and for a few days, so that will help. We also signed up for driver education online, finally. So, he will be working on that and schoolwork since the new school year will start Monday. Hopeful that he handles homebound well and keeps his grades up.

August 29, 2017

- 65 days post diagnosis
- Day 29 of Consolidation

Well, he didn't make counts today, so no chemo this week. This is the chemo hold/break the doc mentioned may be needed. We will check counts again Tuesday to see if they are up enough for chemo.

His Fibrinogen and Antithrombin III counts are low again, so four more units of plasma are on schedule for today.

He started homebound schooling last week. He has a couple of assignments he needs to complete if I can keep him awake long enough to do them. We'll try that again this evening.

Also, we are still in need of donations for the silent auction for the benefit on September 17th. Please consider donating.

September 2, 2017

Please keep Mikey in your thoughts and prayers.

Mom took him to ER earlier due to severe headache and vomiting. They decided to admit him due to dehydration.

They then did MRI to check for blood clots since he has the blood clotting disorder and one of his chemo meds is known to cause clots. They determined there were several clots in the brain so they are starting blood thinners and he will be in hospital until at least Monday.

Their goal is to get his headaches and vomiting under control so he will be more comfortable while the blood thinners dissolve the clots. He will also receive more plasma as well as his chemo meds. Pray for him to feel better soon.

September 19, 2017

The clinic was an easy one today. Only about five hours long.

But it flew by with all the conversations we had with the nurses and the doc. Mikey was quite talkative today.

That's okay, though, that means he was feeling good.

His platelets and RBC were low, so he received one unit of each. I've learned quickly how to tell when he's needing blood product because he gets very pale and tires very easily.

His dose of Lovenox is being lowered a bit and it was explained today that they are working on determining which oral anticoagulant will be best for him. It was also said that he will need to take them for life due to the gene mutation combined with the fact that he has gotten a clot.

He will have another MRI around the first of October to check the clots. Hopefully, his body has been working on dissolving them and they will be smaller.

We also discussed whether to continue the PEG Aspariginase in future treatment. There are three more doses in the treatment protocol. Statistically, this specific protocol has a success rate of about 80-85% and the PEG is a key factor in that.

There is no way to know how much his chances of kicking ALL will decrease if we remove the PEG. However, continuing the PEG, even while on anticoagulants, raises the risk of another clot now that he's clotted once.

What do you do?? I just don't know. Thankful that we have time to think about it at least.

Thursday will be the last chemo treatment of this Consolidation phase. He will have a break from chemo while his numbers recover and will then go on to start Interim Maintenance 1. IM is eight weeks long. The doc says this phase should be easier on him. There will be four hospital stays during IM, each stay lasting three or four days. The chemo will be administered during these stays.

That's all I've got for an update for tonight.

I do want to say one quicker thing... THANK YOU!

Thanks to our wonderful neighbors, who took turns bringing Mikey and me dinner after his first hospital stay. Neighbors who I hadn't ever met or spoke to prior to this. Y'all are awesome.

Thanks to all of you that follow what's going on and continue to pray and keep us in your thoughts, even though you don't personally know us.

Thanks to my boss for being as wonderful as he is. He's stuck with me.

Thanks to my friends. My amazing support system. For always checking in to ask how Mikey is doing and to remind me that you're there when I need you.

We are very blessed with amazing friends that have continuously been by our sides and have gone beyond for us since June 25th, which has in turn brought forward their friends and their friends' friends and so on. I couldn't find the words without breaking down in tears yesterday.

Seeing all y'all there, most strangers to us, there to help and support our boy. It was emotionally overwhelming . Thank you all.

September 26, 2017

"He has Leukemia."

Those are the words I heard three months ago. 13 weeks ago. 93 days ago. 2,232 hours ago. It feels like it's been a lifetime already.

I was instantly mad at those words. I thought, "What!? This chick is crazy! How would you even know that!?! We JUST got here like five seconds ago!"

My next reaction was tears. Lots of tears. There's no way. He isn't bruised up. He isn't sick. He has pain in his side. He's an athlete. He's active all the time. He was just swimming at the lake with his friends the evening before. He just played baseball.

His side hurt—that was it. He must have hurt himself at the lake somehow. He's a healthy kid. Hardly ever gets sick. He just had friends stay the night, maybe they were messing around too rough. His side was hurting!

My husband was at work in New Mexico. I needed to call him ASAP. I needed to tell him to come home; our boy has Leukemia. Cancer.

OMG! OUR BABY HAS CANCER!!!

Everything was a whirlwind from that point forward. There were nurses starting an IV, grabbing blood for labs, getting orders for medications. The resident doc was saying that the oncology doc was going to be coming back up to the hospital to meet us to explain what was going to happen next and that treatment needed to start right away.

My phone was going nuts! For days. The calls, texts, FB messages... Although appreciated it, I couldn't keep up and I couldn't keep my phone charged. I just wanted to scream. I just needed to breathe.

There were what seemed like one hundred medical professionals in and out of the room for the next few days. There was paperwork that needed to be signed, permissions for tests and procedures to check his spinal fluid for leukemia and to take some of his bone marrow. Permissions for sedation and surgery to place his port.

There was a binder. A binder full of valuable information: phone numbers to reach the oncology office, the after-hours pager, the hospital. Information, including side effects, about medications I had never heard of before. Chemotherapy medications. Meds can have some insanely scary side effects! Some can stop his heart, some cause clots, some can make him extremely sick.

I quickly realized that we were about to allow these doctors to poison our son in an attempt to kill the cancer. What is happening!?!? How does this happen? How do you take your seemingly healthy kid in for some sudden pain in his side and he is diagnosed with leukemia?!?

T-cell acute lymphoblastic leukemia (ALL) now controls our lives for the next few years. I had never before heard of ALL specifically. I assumed leukemia was simply a cancer of the blood with a good cure rate. I didn't know there were diverse types of leukemia.

I also assumed chemo was "just a special kind of medicine" used to kill cancer. I had no idea how complex chemotherapy and treatment actually is. No clue how dangerous these medications are. My knowledge of leukemia was based on what I saw and read in *My Sister's Keeper*.

Now that I am a cancer mom, now that I've done some reading up and asked many questions, I can recall symptoms before the side pain. Symptoms that I, not unlike any other parent, didn't really think much of.

Now that I am a cancer mom, I can see how ignorant I was about leukemia prior to Sunday, June 25th, 2017.

November 13, 2017

He is clearing this dose like a rock star y'all!!

Remember, MTX level must be 0.1 or lower to discharge. Labs are drawn every 12 hours post MTX to check the level.

His 42-hour level was 0.52 (down from 1.69 @36) and his 48-hour level was 0.24! Next lab will be at noon and results a couple of hours after that.

Now, I remember from last time not to get too excited about the possibility of getting out of here quickly. I remember he had finally started making progress lowering the MTX level and the next lab it had only dropped like half a point or some ridiculousness.

But I am keeping positive that they will be kicking us out of here Tuesday morning.

Mikey was able to get one of his favorite nurses yesterday! He hasn't had her the last couple of stays. He requested her for today too and got his way. No surprise there.

As I was ready to wrap up this post, Dr. G came in to see Michael, who was still sleeping of course, as he was yesterday too.

Dr. G shook his head and then explained that he knows exactly what is going on here: Baseball players are the most superstitious athletes there are and therefore Mikey obviously does not want anything to do with him until he knows he is for sure getting out of here tomorrow.

We discussed that Mikey has been eating well. In fact, he sent me to Taco Bell at 7:30 last night: after the blood count he decided he was hungry again. Then Dr. G told me the results are looking good. Labs will be drawn again at noon and then not again till the morning.

January 18, 2018

Michael got PEG-Asparginase in clinic today. PEG takes two hours: an hour to infuse, followed by an hour of flushing. This chemotherapy drug is pretty scary for us, as it largely contributed to Mikey's blood clots in his brain. His vitals are monitored closely during infusion due to the serious side effects of PEG.

He also needed plasma today. Two units. His doctors monitor clotting factors regularly, specifically the fibrinogen level. They say it's all about balancing his counts due to his clotting disorder (hyper coagulability) and the chemotherapies. Lovenox works by keeping certain clotting factors at safer levels, and the chemo drugs tend to lower those factors.

We had to switch his nausea medicine back to Zofran for now because Kytril is apparently on backorder. They don't even have the IV form in clinic!

Zofran didn't seem to help during Induction and Consolidation; the Kytril was much better for him. This phase of treatment is a "repeat" of part of Induction and Consolidation, so I sure hope the Zofran helps better this time. Besides, I can manage $6 or so easier than over $100!

We will go back to clinic again Friday for labs and any needed blood product transfusions (probably plasma). He will also stop taking the steroids on Friday. At that point it is expected that his counts will drop again, and he will be neutropenic. Then we wait however long it may take for his counts to come up so that he can move onto the next round (Consolidation repeat) of chemo.

March 13, 2018

Mikey got his monthly pentamidine treatment in clinic today. No chemo today as it was a lab day to check counts.

He needed one unit of platelets and two units of FFP (plasma) today. Since he reacted to either PEG or FFP last week, they premedicated today. Kytril (nausea med) hoping to prevent vomiting after Benadryl, and Benadryl hoping to avoid any reactions.

Poor kid vomited right after they administered the Benadryl and broke out with the hives again.

IV Benedryl is just too much for him to handle, even when it's administered slowly. The hives spread quite a bit this time. Arms, back, neck, belly, face, hands. Red and blotchy. Poor guy.

He's obviously developed a sensitivity to the FFP. It's interesting that you can get/take something over and over with no issues and then suddenly develop a reaction.

Anyway, at least we know now that the hives are a reaction to the FFP, not the PEG.

After a dose of oral Benadryl, we headed home. The hives mostly cleared within a few hours. As of tonight, he still had some blotchiness on his belly and chest, so he took another dose of Benadryl before bed.

He lost another two pounds last week. This is something the docs are keeping an eye on. He hasn't lost a lot, but it has been trending recently.

Although he isn't eating a whole lot these days, he is eating. Sometimes he just feels full quicker or doesn't have much of an appetite.

Next clinic day is Friday, for chemo. Vincristine & IV MTX.

June 25, 2018

One year ago, today our lives were completely changed when we entered the world of childhood cancer.

In the US alone, an estimated 15,000+ children under the age of 20 will be diagnosed with cancer each year. Approximately 1 in every 285 children will be diagnosed with cancer before their 20th birthday and more than 40,000 children undergo treatment for cancer each year.

I've learned a little bit over the last year. I joined several Facebook support groups, followed several children's cancer Facebook pages, and have even met a couple of local kids undergoing treatment. I've seen multiple young lives lost to this monster. Some to the disease itself, some due to complications of treatment. Babies, toddlers, teenagers.

THIS SHOULD NOT BE HAPPENING!

August 12, 2018

September is Childhood Cancer Awareness Month:

We're just over 14 months into this unwelcome journey. Since Mikey's diagnosis, I've followed several childhood cancer Facebook pages and groups. I follow many other kiddos who have been invaded by cancer. I read their parents' posts about their journey. I've cried tears of joy for those sharing a happy moment that they didn't think would ever be. And I've cried many, many tears of pain for the ones who have had to sit and watch their babies leave this world.

Childhood cancer is the leading cause of death by disease in children under the age of nineteen in the US.

I was surprised to learn so much of what I've learned in the last 14 months.

- They say pediatric cancer is rare, yet it doesn't seem rare to me at all!! It feels like it is everywhere & I was just ignorantly oblivious to it prior to June 25th, 2017.

- Every year, an estimated 250,000+ new cases of cancer affect children under the age of 20 **worldwide.**

- **One in 285** children in the U.S. will be diagnosed with cancer by the time they are 20 years old.

- Childhood cancer is not just one disease. It is made up of twelve major types and over one hundred subtypes!

- And the chemotherapy drugs... They are awful! And the side effects are **tremendous.** Did you know that most chemotherapy drugs were developed for adults?

- Did you know that only 4% of federal government cancer research goes to study pediatric cancer? You read that right, 4%! Just four pennies on every dollar! No exaggeration. How is this even possible?

    More than 95% of childhood cancer survivors will have significant, long-lasting health-related issue(s) by the time they are 45 years of age due to the side effects of either cancer or the result of its treatment.
    Childhood cancer research is vastly and consistently underfunded!

    All I ask of you is that you share the posts about pediatric cancer. Help spread awareness.

October 29, 2019
    Today is day one of the seventh cycle of maintenance.
    Mikey's counts are slowly improving. His ANC (germ fighting cells) is 980 today, so it is still low-ish but not severely low. His platelet count is still

down, eighty something, but getting there. Seventy-five is the minimum required count to be able to have his LP.

We were asked if we wanted to have a bone marrow aspiration done while we were there for the LP. It was something the docs talked about doing if his counts were still low, but they feel good about the improvement in his ANC, so they let us decide. Michael felt it wasn't necessary right now, so we declined.

He got his Vincristine in clinic through his port, before going over to the hospital for his procedure. The LP went smoothly; they obtained their two samples of CSF and injected the methotrexate.

His blood pressure was dropping from the propofol, so they monitored him extra in recovery today. It's a known side effect of propofol but has only recently become "a thing" with the boy. Once his BP came up some and was steady, they were able to get us on our way.

Doc told us to resume oral chemo at home, but at half the dosage he was taking prior to his counts dropping. He also wants his counts checked again in two weeks and possibly every two weeks continually until his counts are up and stable again (which helps this momma breathe just a little bit easier).

October 2, 2018

Today was a bit unusual. There were some minor procedure changes for accessing his port in clinic, and the SPU was so busy that they did his LP in the pre-op room instead of the procedure room.

There was a new anesthesia doc in there today. She likes to use ketamine with the usual propofol for sedation. She explained that while propofol lowers heart rate, breathing rate, and blood pressure, ketamine brings it up. Mikey's never had ketamine before, so I wasn't sure what to expect.

Everything went well. The LP was quick and easy. One stick as it should be. They didn't rush us out of recovery this time. He woke up on his own but seemed kind of spacey. He wasn't liking the way the ketamine was making him feel while waking up. He had a challenging time seeing straight and said he felt drugged. This continued for a little while. He's made it clear that he does not want it again in the future!

Back in clinic he got his chemo (vincristine) and pentamidine. He usually gets the Pentam through inhalation, but he got it through his port today. I'd say about halfway or so through the Pentam, he began coughing quite a bit and became very phlegmy. Then his lips and around his eyes began to tingle. His lips swelled and his face got red.

We can now add pentamidine to his growing list of allergies . Benadryl was given, and his vitals monitored for a bit until the reaction subsided. He will go back to taking the Bactrim in its place.

They also gave him some morphine to help with his knee pain. I assume that the nurses aggravated his knees when they bent them up during his LP because he was having a lot of pain when he woke up in recovery.

As far as his knees are concerned, there is fluid on both. The left is worse than the right. The knee issues could be from the steroids as they are known to cause osteoarthritis in the larger joints, or it could be that he injured himself during workouts in school. We've got an MRI scheduled for tomorrow and, with any luck, an ortho consult.

His counts seem to be handling chemo well so far. His platelet count came up to 107! Three digits, y'all!! That was a 30,000-point jump from two weeks ago.

Dr. G increased his oral chemo slightly. Now he will take a total of five whole mercaptopurine tablets a week instead of three, and five pills a month of methotrexate instead of four. Baby steps.

Hopefully, his counts continue to do well so they can get him up to his required dosage.

In two weeks, we will go back to clinic to check counts. The day before that, Mikey will have another MRI done on his brain. It's been almost a year since his last MRI that showed his clots were gone.

He's been getting headaches caused by light. Bright, flashing, or sudden. Sometimes from watching tv or being on a computer. Last week he got a headache after his niece shook a glow stick around in a dark room.

This creates a bit of concern.

I think that's about all I have for today. I'll let y'all know what we find out about his knees in a couple of days.

May 24, 2019

Today is day 688 since diagnosis. Day 334 of LTM & day eighty-four of the fourth cycle. 518 more days to go!

Today Michael had another lumbar puncture/spinal tap with intrathecal methotrexate in the hospital's special procedures unit and then went back to the clinic for IV chemo—vincristine via his port.

His counts are still doing quite well. (If y'all remember, his platelets had a pretty tough time recovering during treatment last year, which put him on a chemo hold for something like 72 days. When he finally made counts again, we jumped right into Long Term Maintenance on an exceptionally low dose of oral chemo.)

We are now almost a year into LTM, with gradual dosage increases and no other chemo holds.

Dr. McGregor decided today to increase his 6MP dosage to his full required dose. He will remain taking a lower dosage of the oral methotrexate for now. There's still plenty of time to gradually jump that up to the full required dose.

He's got a job now, which keeps him on his feet a lot, so his knees have been yelling at him and he's been tired. But he's been feeling fairly good for the most part. If y'all haven't looked at the pics from prom, go check them out. He looked SO handsome and healthy and just like a regular teenage boy at his prom.

Today, we were introduced to the Beads of Courage program. I've heard a little about the beads before, but McLane's didn't participate until now. There is a bead given for each experience or accomplishment during treatment, such as bone marrow aspirate, LP, port access, chemo infusion, hospital admission and discharge, end of treatment, and more. We're obviously behind with the boys' collection at the moment.

He received a few today, but I have a lot of looking back to do (thank goodness I keep this page) to list each and every "thing" I can recall, collecting his beads. It's a neat program. He also received a beautiful hand-crafted wooden container for his beads! Folks make these in all different shapes, colors, and designs and donate them to the children's hospitals for their Beads of Courage programs. Such a great program!

That's about all I have to share for today. Tomorrow, we must be in Temple again for his follow up appointment with the knee surgeon. Positive thoughts are always appreciated.

August 11, 2019

Tomorrow is surgery. We must check in at 5 a.m. That's much earlier than I'd hoped for, but better to be first rather than last.

The plan was to go to clinic beforehand so they could access his port for surgery. He will only allow the nurses at the clinic to access him. When I told him what time we have to be at the hospital, he said they would have to do an IV because they're not accessing his port.

He's nervous about surgery, but mostly worried about the immense pain he is expecting. Hopefully, the cleanout won't be as in-depth as the left knee was and he won't be in quite as much pain.

I know he would rather his initial surgeon be the one doing this surgery.

October 3, 2019

The boy had his monthly clinic appointment on Tuesday.

He had another new-to-us nurse. She was an oncology nurse at Memorial for several years before coming to clinic last month. Y'all know he greatly dislikes having someone new access his port. He just laid there & didn't really say a word. She did great, of course. Got it first try with perfect blood return. He said he wasn't anxious, but his face sure said he was.

His labs looked good. His counts continue to stay steady so there will not be any changes to his dosage. He got the usual vincristine infusion through his port, and we were done. Oh, and he got his flu shot too!

He took his eleven tablets of methotrexate & his 6MP before bed. He was so drained after all that chemo on Tuesday that he stayed home from school on Wednesday too. His next visit in four weeks will be day one of Cycle 7 of Maintenance and will include an LP.

As of today, it has been 830 days since he was diagnosed with ALL. He has 375 days left of treatment. A year goes by rather quickly, so I bet before we know it, he will be done with active treatment. Of course, he will continue to be monitored for recurrence and late-term effects of treatment for quite some time. Then, there is long-term follow-up care, which should continue for the rest of his life.

I already silently stress about the "what ifs;" I can't imagine how it will be after treatment ends.

January 4, 2020
Day 933.
In clinic for chemo and an LP today. We talked more with the doc about his knees and the hope to get them replaced sooner rather than later. She plans to talk to a bone doctor from McLane's about seeing the boy. We talked some more about pain management, but he doesn't want to take anything for the pain.

The Hem/Onc clinic is beginning to integrate counseling—something that is long overdue in my opinion. A cancer diagnosis is **huge**. It's life-altering. It completely changes everything going forward. Add to that, being a teenager.

We met the doctor, and he was genuinely nice, young, and chill. I don't think it even felt like a doctor/patient meeting.

Although I think he's handled these last two-plus years with amazing strength and positivity, there were definitely times throughout his treatment that I worried about his mental health.

Concerned about depression or anger. Concerned about his self-esteem and his dwindling friendships.

Neither of us feel he necessarily needs counseling at this point; he's practically a pro now. But it's great to know the option is available if needed. After all, he has a lot of changes coming his way this year!

So, next on the list is to get these knees replaced. How fantastic it would be for him to be able to walk across that stage on May 28th without any pain!

January 28, 2020

Update from yesterday:

I got a call Friday evening from Michael's oncologist letting me know that he spoke with the orthopedic surgeon they're recommending, who agreed to see Michael. It was an "FYI, be ready because it can be as early as Monday" call.

Well, that call came early this morning with a request to be in Temple for a 2 p.m. appointment! So, here we go! Hang tight with me, there were many large medical terms used that I don't remember lol.

They took some new X-rays and examined his knees. He showed us the pictures and pointed out the areas of collapse. We discussed the medical details pertaining to his diagnosis of acute lymphoblastic leukemia 2017 & avascular necrosis in 2018. We talked about the arthroscopic procedures he had in February and August of 2019 to clean up the broken bone and cartilage fragments that were causing his knees to get stuck.

Then we talked about the available options.

1) I cannot recall the name of the procedure, but they basically drill multiple small holes into the bone to stimulate new bone/cartilage growth. This was mentioned to us early on but quickly taken off the table as an option for him. The initial doc was concerned about unintentionally causing fractures since his AVN is so severe. Dr. Ward explained today that he doesn't think this procedure would be helpful to Michael either.

2) Bone grafting surgery. This was the preference of the first orthopedic doctor we saw. For this they take cadaver bone and connect it to his bone so that it fuses & creates healthy bone. Of course, there are risks to surgery and we are not sure how much bone is available to fuse a graft.

3) his final option is total knee replacement surgery. They can last 20 years or more but will need to be replaced again in the future. So, we talked about the risks of surgery again, adding in his immunodeficiency due to chemotherapy. But in the end, this surgery appears to be his best option.

The visit went well, and the doctor was wonderful. He took his time with us, explaining and answering questions. He even provided us with his personal cell number (and told the boy to call ANYTIME he feels he needs to, day/night/weekends)! But we did not get the answer for which we were hoping.

We were not told "We can do this now. Let's get it set up." We were told that the best way to do this to get the absolute best results, is to wait until he finishes treatment. *Enter tears of disappointment & frustration at this point*

He made clear to us that he was in no way dismissing Michael's pain. He explained that his biggest concern is the risk of infection. Think about it: your body needs germ-fighting cells to fight and knock out infection. Chemo beats on and knocks out your germ fighters. So, it would not be possible to finish treatment if he got an infection.

Michael is understandably concerned about just how bad his knees will continue to get over the next nine months. Nine months is a long time. What if he ends up not being able to walk at all before October? But what if he got an infection after surgery? What if the leukemia came back because he couldn't finish treatment because he got an infection after surgery? There are just so many "what ifs."

In the end, everything the doc said makes sense and if he isn't comfortable with surgery during treatment, then we wait. I was personally incredibly pleased with him, his honesty, and his obvious care about what is best for my boy.

We will follow up with visits every four to six weeks to allow him the opportunity to follow Michael until the end of treatment and the time allowed for the surgery.

I ask today, that you send positive vibes our boy's way. Some positive thoughts that he doesn't suffer with too much terrible pain between now and end of treatment and for his feelings of disappointment and frustration to be replaced with the vision of immense success he will have with his brand-new knees later on this year!

February 11, 2020
Today is day 961. Nine hundred sixty-one.

- 961 days since diagnosis.
- 959 days since the first infusion of chemotherapy.
- 932 days in remission.
- 607 days since beginning the Maintenance phase of treatment.
- The 35th day of Cycle 8 of Maintenance.
- 242 days until what we thought was the end of treatment.
- **Today Mikey's treatment was extended by 168 days.** The disappointment was real & so the tears.

It was recommended that we add two additional cycles of maintenance treatment, pushing his EOT to about mid-March or so of 2021. Because of AVN. Because he had to stop taking steroids. Steroids are such an important part of treatment. I have worried about what the outcome will be without being able to take the steroids.

But what do you do?

The steroids caused osteonecrosis in his knees, and they would have continued to cause more damage, even in other joints. So, you stop them.

There is no data that says adding these extra two cycles of treatment will indeed prevent relapse. Hell, the entire treatment for ALL is trial and error. Nothing is guaranteed.

But if something is suggested and recommended, that is what we are going to do. Like the boy said this morning, "What if I don't do the extra cycles and I relapse? I would hate to feel like I maybe could've prevented it by doing the two extra cycles."

So, the knees are put off for even longer now, which is a big, big deal for him. But "what's the point of new knees if I relapsed?"

I know that we all feel bombarded with the terrible things in life sometimes. That's why there are well-known sayings like "when it rains it pours" or "He doesn't give you more than you can handle," right? But it is just SO stinking hard not to feel angry. I hate that my boy is hurting (in many ways), and I can't do a single thing to make it better.

June 9, 2021

Look at these counts.

For the first time in FOUR YEARS the boy's counts are "perfect."

Every month I silently worry. Without chemo keeping leukemia away and with four weeks between appointments, the anxiety gets me. That will probably never go away.

But this!

November 3, 2021

I have slacked off with updates these last couple of months. Life has been... well, rough here lately.

But the boy is doing wonderfully!

- He attends in person classes twice a week & virtual classes twice a week. The semester is nearly finished already!
- He finished PT for his left knee at the end of September and has started playing golf a bit again.
- He has chosen to wait a while for the next knee surgery.
- Right now, any pain and discomfort are manageable, or I should say "bearable" because he doesn't really take anything for pain at all. His surgeon made a move to another facility, so when the time comes, we hope to be able to see him in Waco rather than having to travel.

Mikey has gone to the clinic on his own twice now. Only because I was out of town last month dealing with my mother's passing and I had a pre-op appointment yesterday. It's a tough transition for *me*, but he's perfectly OK with it. But his labs continue to look great!

That's all I have for now. Next clinic visit is in four weeks!

March 29, 2022

Today marks ONE FULL YEAR of being OFF TREATMENT!

The emotions I feel today are just as intense as they were when he rang the bell last year. I am so ridiculously proud of this boy!

Mikey had his monthly visit to the oncologist on Monday. His counts still look good, and he is feeling well overall. He has "graduated" to oncology visits every two months now. That's a long time in between visits, which is overwhelming, but he has done well, and this is the next step in after treatment care.

He got a job at a local convenience store a few weeks ago! Going to school and working takes a little getting used to, but he is managing well. He is happy to be working and making some money. They do a little bit of everything in a shift (register, stocking, cleaning, etc.), so he is constantly on his feet, which has had him in pain.

Some of that pain is from using muscles he doesn't use often; however, some of it is joint pain in his knees, shoulders, and hips. Knee pain is to be expected due to the AVN, but the hip and shoulder pain are new.

His orthopedic surgeon did tell us that he could very well have AVN in his other joints based on the severity of his knees, but he wasn't having pain in any other joints back then. We talked about making an appointment with the orthopedic doc if we need to, but he doesn't want to right now. So, we will see how things go and how he feels as the days go by.

Oh, and he has a birthday coming up at the end of the month–the big 2-0!! Here's to YOU kid! You deserve nothing but the best for your future!

June 25, 2022

Five years ago today, I made a post, sitting in Premier ER and Urgent Care, that I had taken the boy in to be checked out and hoped it wasn't anything serious. I had no idea the journey that was upon us.

I had taken Mikey to the ER because he had been up all night with severe pain up his left side and neck. I was thinking he had hurt himself jumping with his friends at Tonkawa Falls during the days before.

An exam discovered his spleen was swollen. Then we discussed some other symptoms he'd been experiencing over the recent days: a mild sore throat, feeling overly tired and achy. The doctor was thinking mono and he ran labs and ordered scans.

After several hours of being in the ER, scans confirmed an enlarged spleen & blood work showed a WBC of over 220,000 (double-checked). I was asked to choose a children's hospital to be transferred to for further testing.

He mentioned that Mikey's symptoms could sometimes be linked to leukemia or lymphoma, but that just sounded so absurd that I didn't give it a second thought. Denial began right away, I suppose.

I chose McLane Children's Hospital in Temple because it's closest to home and no one has time for traffic to Dallas or Austin. Yes, that was the reasoning for my choice and thankfully I've had no regrets on that decision!

McLane's arranged for transport while we waited for them for what felt like an eternity. I followed the ambulance to Temple, through a backed-up I-35. I remember feeling anxious and very frustrated with the ridiculous amount of traffic on a Sunday evening. When I finally got into the ER, they were already bringing Mikey up to a room, so I was asked to wait until they got him settled.

When I was finally sent up to see him, I walked into the room, and he was in the bed. A young doctor was sitting on the couch beside the bed. She introduced herself as the resident doctor and asked, "Do you know why you're here?"

I replied, "He was sent here for more testing because he apparently has an enlarged spleen..."

That's when our entire world as we knew it came crashing down on us with her response, in these EXACT words: **"He has leukemia."**

My heart immediately sank. There he was, my baby, lying in this hospital bed with his head down and tears falling. His whole life just came to a screeching halt. I remember crying and thinking there had to be some kind of mistake.

We hadn't even gotten a glimpse of what this really meant yet. This journey was not easy.

Despite the emotions.

Despite the awful side effects of chemo that he had: blood clots in his brain, excruciating pain in his legs that kept him awake at night, AVN in both knees, headaches, nausea, vomiting, diarrhea, sores in his mouth and down his throat, all around feeling like garbage.

Despite all that he lost: missing a true high school experience, the opportunity to play Cougar baseball and to continue ball into college. Through all of that, he pushed through EVERY SINGLE DAY.

He is literally BADASS. His strength and determination never faltered. He is MY HERO and there are no words that could ever express how proud I am to be his mother.

This year, he wants to recognize today, which took me by surprise. "It is part of my history at the end of the day." He's right. So tonight, we will have dinner together at his request.

September 12, 2022

It's been a long while since I've posted. No news is good news, right? The boy is doing pretty good overall. His bi-monthly oncology appointments continue. They have gone well, and his lab results continue to look great!

He does have an upcoming CT for a lump that he found recently. He initially saw our family doctor when he first discovered it. She felt that it wasn't anything serious but said it would need imaging. She thought it best to refer him to a general surgeon to handle that. I mentioned that I would prefer him to see a specialist within Baker, Scott, and White hospital system since he was already an established patient there, but she assured me that this doctor was wonderful (and local), and she trusted him very much.

It took a couple of weeks to get in to see the specialist, and when Mikey met with him, the boy was not impressed in the least bit. The doctor wasn't very personable and pretty much rushed the appointment. He told Mikey that he was ordering a CT and that he would want to remove the lump, due to his medical history.

I want to recommend surgery without even knowing what it was unnecessary, but we were rolling with it for the moment. The CT was scheduled for last Friday, but I cancelled it after Mikey saw his oncologist last week.

Dr. M was unaware of the lump (he found it after his July clinic visit) until Mikey mentioned it at the clinic. He said no one had let him know about it, which was disappointing because he kept our family doctor completely in the loop throughout Mikey's treatment. He said that he wouldn't want to see him have surgery that isn't necessary. He asked that *he* schedule the CT and refer Mikey to their surgeon, if needed.

Of course, we would prefer that anyway.

So, the CT is scheduled for the 28th and then he will follow up with Dr. M after that.

His knees are still a daily issue to some extent.

He saw the orthopedic surgeon in mid-July because he was contemplating moving forward with the graft on his right knee, but he had injured his left knee shortly before his appointment (the one he already had the graft on), so they sent him for an MRI on that one first.

Overall, the left knee looks the same as it did post-surgery, but his meniscus needs some repairing. He has decided to put off any surgery as long as he possibly can, so they have opted to try knee injections to see if that helps for now. His first appointment for that will be this week.

I'll post again soon!

January 4, 2023

Quick update on the boy. His counts are perfect again! He's done so great since finishing treatment.

I went to clinic with him this time to get some clarity on his having to leave pediatrics and begin seeing a new oncologist.

Dr. M explained that the necessity for him to move out of pediatrics is due to McLane's not having the right doctors available to treat him as an adult, if needed. The further out we get from treatment, the less likely relapse is, but **if** he were to relapse or end up with a secondary cancer, he would need to be treated and cared for by adult care doctors.

Dr. M will get a referral, likely to BSW oncology group here in Waco, and Mikey will make the switch this summer.

He will see Dr. M just two more times: in March, which marks two years of treatment, at which time he will move to appointments every three months. And then for the last time in June.

I think it's going to be a tough transition, emotionally. Adult care is nothing like the pediatric care we've received for almost six years. It's not like anything I've experienced before.

There's a bond there. They chit-chat and talk about sports and life. He truly cares about what's happening in the boy's life and what/how he's doing. And he has been with us since right after diagnosis.

Case #26:

Robin & Husband, Mike's, Melanoma

I've known Robin for several years. She was a remarkably successful franchisee for one of our brands. I met her husband, Mike, on one of the trips we had where only the best of the best were invited to attend.

In fact, she was named Franchisee of the Year for that brand in the past couple years.

After I posted my message on Facebook in January, I learned that Mike was diagnosed with Melanoma. I interviewed Robin and learned this incredibly sad story. The good news is they have a wonderful doctor, great support system as well as prayer warriors.

December, 2021. Mike and Robin, from Jersey, are in Hilton Head at a great resort with Mike's brother, Tom, and his family from Florida. Wonderful way to relax and have family time between the Christmas and New Year's holidays.

On December 30th, Mike and Robin were heading down to see Mike's cousin in Jekyll Island ... a trip that was long overdue. Mike and Robin were really excited to see him and his wife.

That morning, Robin heard Mike let out a scream in the shower. When she arrived at the bathroom, he was bent down, looking up at the ceiling and shaking. She gets Tom and he runs into the bathroom to see if he can help. Mike isn't responsive. Emergency medics were there in no time.

Mike wasn't responsive in the ER for over 30 minutes. Of course, they had no idea what it could be. Doctors thought he might have suffered a stroke.

After initial scans showed older spots on his brain, doctors asked Robin if Mike suffered any head injuries. By now, Mike was able to respond that he never had any head injuries before he met Robin, and none since. He had two additional seizures while in the ER.

Mike went for additional testing. He was moved into a quiet, private room. Tom had to wait in the outside waiting room due to COVID restrictions. After a period of time, the nursing staff allowed Tom to join Robin in the room with Mike. The doctors returned and reported to Robin and Tom that the scans showed Mike had tumors in his brain (which caused the seizures) lungs, liver, colon and under his left arm. It also appeared that lymph nodes were swollen. Considering the one of the larger tumors was located in the colon, they were convinced had colon cancer. They biopsied the tumor under the arm as it was the easiest to get to. The ER doctor advised it would take three to five days to receive the results of the biopsy.

Robin became agitated with herself. Mike was supposed to get a colonoscopy when he was fifty. He didn't. He cancelled three appointments, and she didn't stay on his butt to make sure he got one. Now, 13 years later, they were going through this.

The doctors at Hilton Head advised Robin to make an appointment with an oncologist as soon as possible as Mike had Stage IV colon cancer. It was critical for Mike to be seen ASAP. With COVID restrictions, appointments with specialist doctors were exceedingly difficult to obtain.

Using her connections back home, Robin got a referral to a local colorectal surgeon at a cancer hospital in New Jersey. He made an appointment with an oncologist for Jan 6th and asked Robin to bring all documents to him once they arrived back home.

On January 2nd, Robin, Mike, and Tom made the 12-hour drive back to Jersey. Robin and Mike were grateful to have family with them during this stressful heath crisis.

Five days later, the biopsy results came back from Hilton Head advising that Mike's cancer was not colon cancer, it was Stage IV melanoma that had metastasized. The colon cancer doctor referred him to a doctor who specialized in melanoma and a radiology oncologist who specialized in brain tumors.

The decision Robin and Mike had to make was whether they should go to a cancer hospital in New York, Philadelphia or stay closer to home in New Jersey which was 20 minutes from their home. They were told the protocol of care will be the same no matter where they went but they may have access to clinical trials at different institutions should Mike be deemed an ideal candidate to participate in them if needed. After meeting with the local oncologist, they opted to stay local. They trusted this oncology team and knew they needed to work with an oncologist they trusted.

While this was all happening, Robin was dealing with lingering personal fears. Lung cancer runs in the family. She was a smoker years ago and both her parents smoked for years. Although she quit, she has fears of getting it herself. Ten years ago, she had a lung cancer screening to see if she might have it. The results of that screening showed a nodule on her lung. She was referred to a pulmonologist who suggested a biopsy.

Robin believes in holistic medicine, so she opted to not get the biopsy. Instead, she consulted a local radiologist. He advised "If you were my wife, I would suggest you see a thoracic surgeon and let him decide the path." She went to a thoracic surgeon who suggested that they watch it every year.

Both Mike and Robin loved Mike's doctor. Dr. W was direct, and while new to their local hospital, she had overseen clinical trials in her former role. The first thing Dr, W urged them to do was to get rid of the brain tumors. A radiologist took care of this in January 2022.

Chemo doesn't work to fight melanoma. Immunotherapy is the recommended treatment, but it comes with side effects. Colitis, arthritis, and other 'itis' issues.

Mike did get colitis requiring hospital stays, one lasting 45 days in the Summer. He had already been to the ER in April and May several times. He dropped over twenty pounds, and there was concern that he wasn't "meaty" enough to endure what lay ahead.

Things were busy at home. Robin had her business to run. Their daughter was planning a 2023 wedding. The doctor urged the family to consider a wedding sooner for obvious reasons. Everyone wanted Mike to feel good enough to walk his daughter down the aisle and celebrate her marriage.

The kids had two ceremonies – one for immediate family only in August. In October they had the "happily ever after party" for 150 people. Both were wonderful and appreciated by all.

Robin had been in the medical device world for 21 years before making the decision to own her own franchise. She knew the importance of having a hands-on advocate. She could follow up on the medicines Mike was prescribed and why those were the meds that he needed.

She also could choose other caretakers he would need – like a wound care specialist. This person might have saved his life as during the 45-day hospital day. He had an allergic reaction to blood thinners that caused two large wounds on his abdomen. Robin knew the treatment recommended by the dermatologist at the hospital was wrong and could cause harm to Mike. Robin requested a wound care consultation. The wound care nurse agreed with Robin and treated Mike differently than originally recommended by the dermatologist. The wounds took months to heal, were very painful and added days to Mike's hospital stay.

Robin reached out to friends and family about visiting Mike. She created a visitation schedule to help keep Mike's spirits up and to bring him fattening food to help him gain weight – vanilla milkshakes and mashed potatoes were two of Mike's favorites.

When Mike returned home, Robin was on a mission to help Mike regain the weight he lost and to add more weight just in case he got sick again. She made sure he consumed 3500 calories a day. He regained twenty pounds plus an additional fifteen.

He had a great late summer and fall. He was handling all of the medicines and feeling better. Everything was going according to the doctor's plans.

Mike started having pain in his rib area just after Christmas. As they moved into 2023 the goal for Mike and Robin was to find the right "cocktail of medicines" that will help him feel the most comfortable. This is exceedingly difficult to find what will work the best as everyone reacts differently to pain medicine.

Over the past several months some of the tumors have been shrinking. Others are stable. The cocktails needed for this might be necessary for years. Their doctor's #1 goal is to help Mike simply feel better. He hurts all the time. Extremely hard on Mike, Robin, and the family as much as one wants to empathize, no one understands the pain like Mike.

Robin wonders what is going through Mike's mind. I imagine it is what I wondered what was going through Mary Kay's mind when we both thought I had cancer. Like Mike, I knew what I was thinking and was afraid to hear what my wife was worried about.

Robin is a stress eater. She knows if Mike can be cured, she will lose the fifteen pounds she put on since he was diagnosed. This, plus the challenges of owning your own business, equal exhaustion. Still, she goes on . . . one day at a time . . . she is not letting him go.

Looking back both tried to figure out how Mike got melanoma. He doesn't have a melanoma mole on his body. They learned that one can get melanoma through their eyes, mouth, and ears. As a kid Mike was a lifeguard and a competitive swimmer. He was one of the top breast strokers in New Jersey. One of his best friends mentioned that he always had blisters on his lips, always in the sun, either life guarding or swimming.

Robin still has the worries of lung cancer. Last summer she met with her dermatologist, then thoracic surgeon, to continue her quest to stay healthy. The dermatologist removed a pre-melanoma mole in May. The Thoracic surgeon did a whole-body PET scan as her lung nodule had grown. She was and is cancer free.

Of course, she told Mike about it – but after the fact. She knew he had had enough to worry about then.

Mike and Robin are both Catholic and believe in the power of prayer. They have a huge Prayer Warrior network praying for Mike. Mary Kay and I are now part of this network.

Robin's concluding thoughts were about testing and doing what doctors want us to do.

If your doctor recommends you do a coloscopy. Do it. Today. Don't wait.

Diagnosed

- If you are a smoker, do the scan to see if you might have lung cancer.
- Did you love to tan when you were a kid? Get a dermatologist.
- Early detection can save a life.

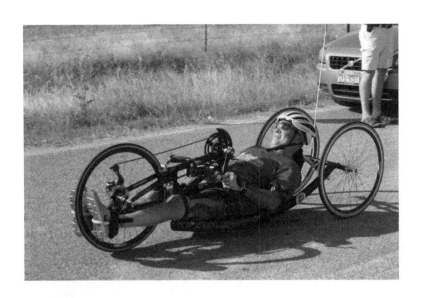

Doug from "Doug's Story – A True Jesus Warrior"

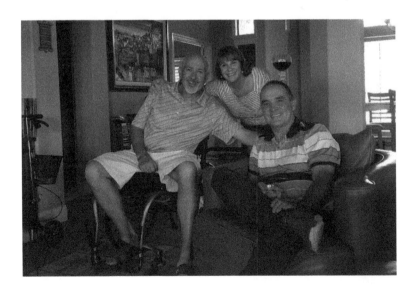

Doug & Wife, Liz, from "Doug from Doug's Story – a True Jesus Warrior"

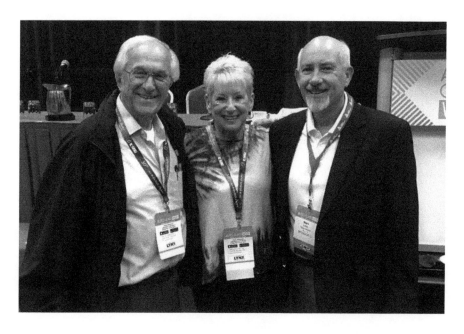

Nancy and husband, Dick, from "Nancy–Lung Cancer"

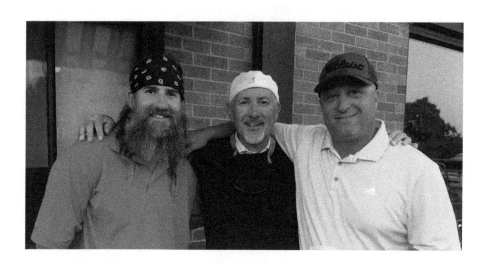

Son, Tom, from "Jerry–Pancreatic Cancer & a Lesson" with son, Andy, on Left

Runaways can still find help

Dear Abby: In the summer of 1974, I was a runaway teenage girl from Kansas living on the streets of Las Vegas. A Good Samaritan who called himself "Nard" befriended me.

He showed me a column you had written about

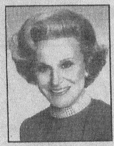

DEAR ABBY

ABIGAIL
VAN BUREN

Operation Peace of Mind, a program that allowed runaway kids to communicate with their families without disclosing their whereabouts. Operation Peace of Mind's philosophy worked for me. It got me out of a dangerous situation and back home where I belonged. My family and I will always be grateful to Operation Peace of Mind, to Nard and to you, Abby, for making this information available.

Does Operation Peace of Mind or anything similar still exist? Thank you, 22 wonderful years later. — **Janet Ramos, Corte Madera, Calif.**

Dear Janet: It's gratifying to know that you received the help you needed so long ago.

Although Operation Peace of Mind no longer exists, the need for such programs has not diminished. The streets of major cities all across America are often the only "home" young runaways are able to find.

Fortunately, another organization that helps runaway and homeless youths, and those who are considering leaving home, does exist.

The National Runaway Switchboard is a toll-free, 24-hour hotline that provides confidential crisis intervention and referrals for youth in crisis and their families. By calling (800) 621-4000, young people nationwide who are stranded on the streets can be referred to a nearby shelter where they can spend the night safely. Teens can also receive crisis counseling, be referred to community-based organizations, and/or have a message delivered (in confidence) or a conference call to their families.

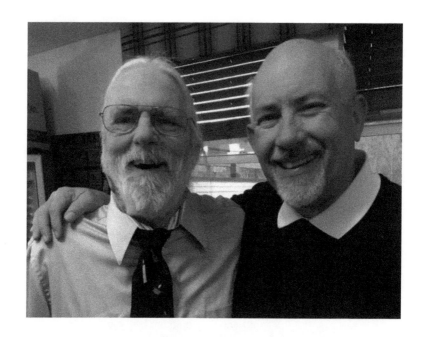

Nard from "Nard – ALS & a Love Story"

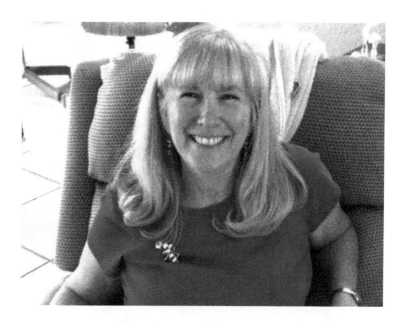

MK's sister, Marti from "Marti Single Mastectomy & Possible Lung Cancer"

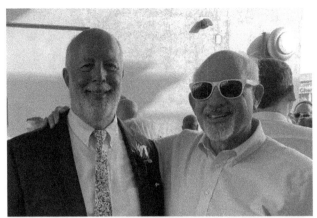

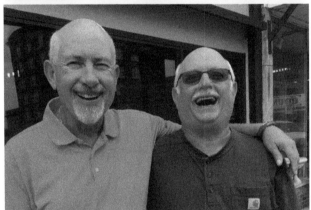

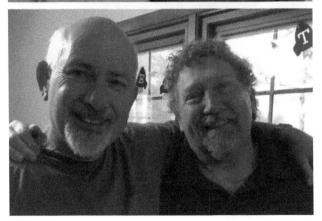

Friends Greg, (top) David, and Chris (bottom)

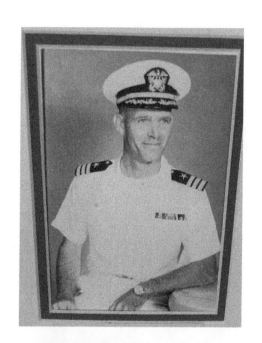

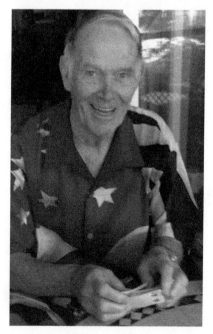

MK's dad Bill Shields

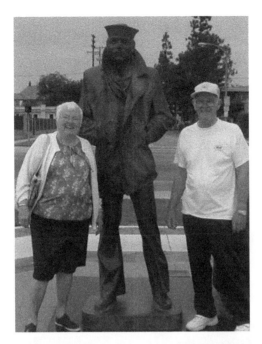

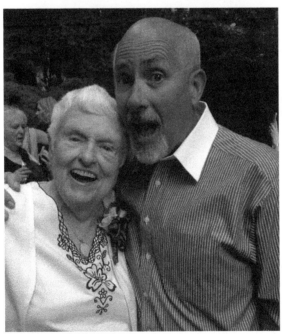

MK's mom Ruth Shields

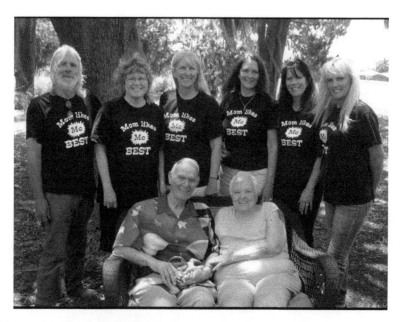

Mom and Dad with Shields kids by age Nard, MK, Marti, Micki, Meg, and Miriam

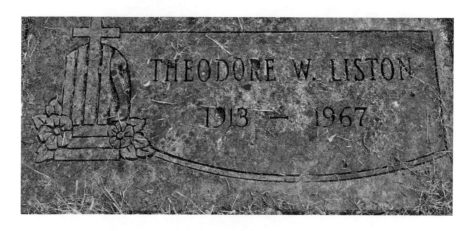

Honoring my dad – what a splendid example for me

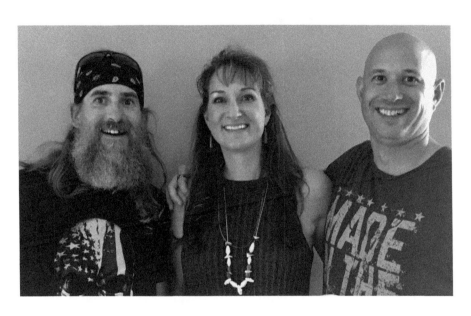

The kids–Andy, Jae, and Marcus

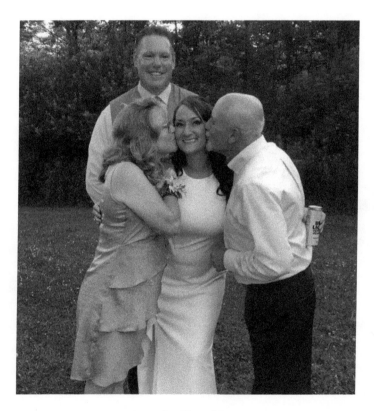

Jae and Jeff's wedding

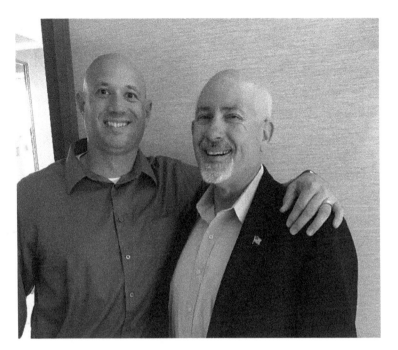

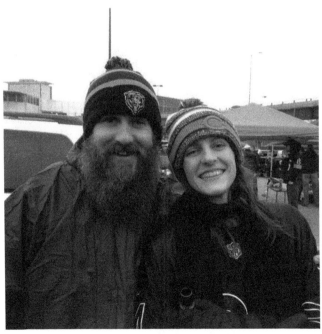

Marcus and Andy and Sarah

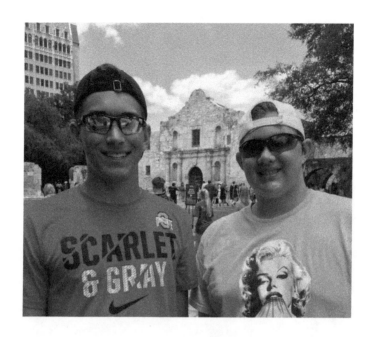

The two oldest grandsons at the Alamo

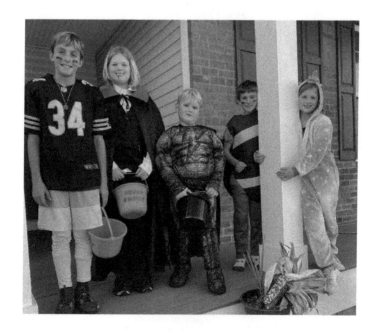

Five youngest at our house for Halloween

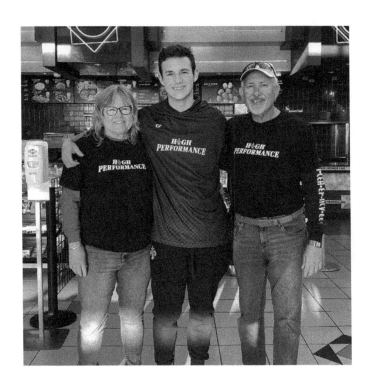

The third oldest grand at his volleyball tournament

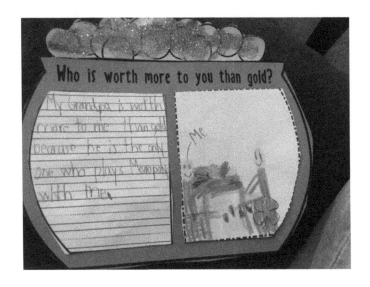

The best thing about being a grandpa is notes like this!

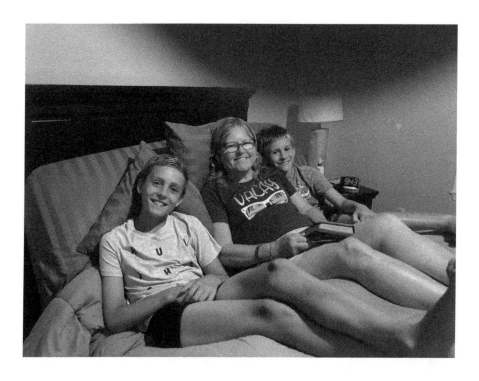

Grammie loves to read Bible stories when boys sleep over

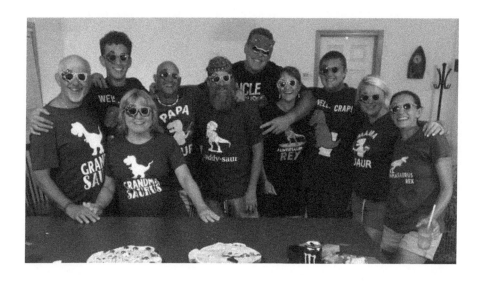

Vacation with the fam at the beach

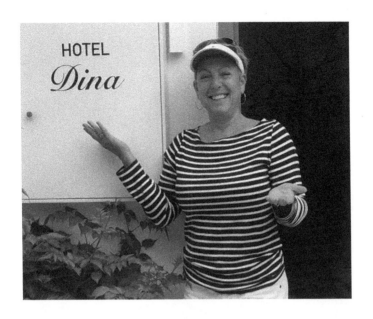

Vacationing in Greece with Dina. Not really her hotel but we did work for her company!

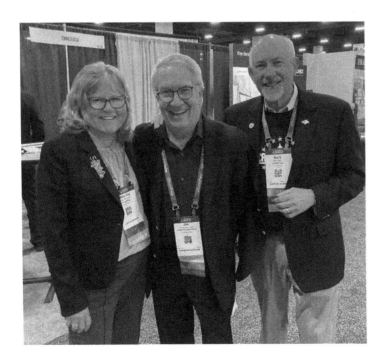

With Joe B

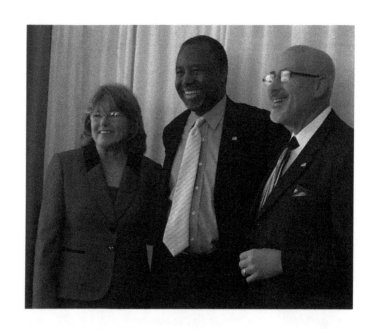

Lunch with Ben Carson when he ran for US President

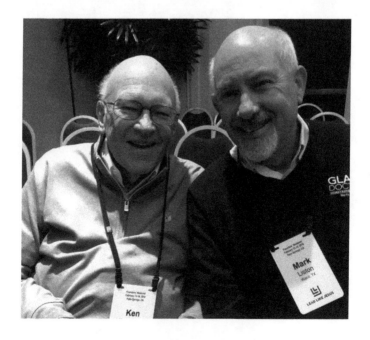

With Ken Blanchard at Lead Like Jesus event

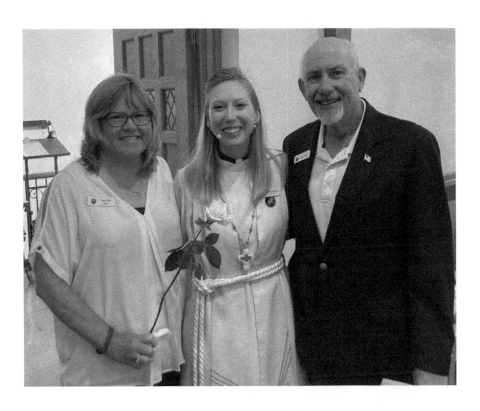

With our Pastor Marissa on Mother's Day

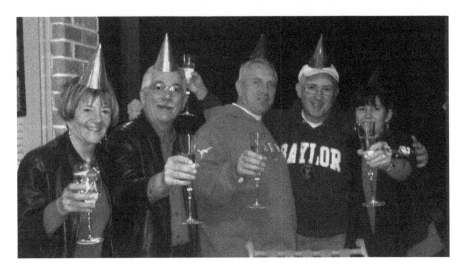

Our Annual NY Eve with Mary and Will in Waco. Joined that year by Mary's parents from Paris

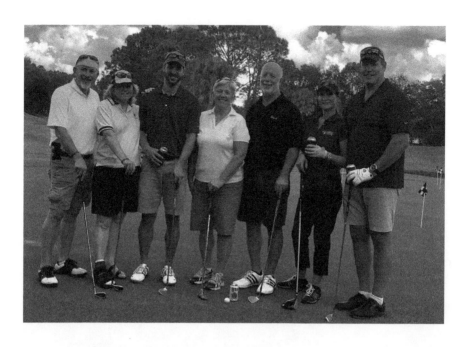

Our annual Christmas golf event with Greg's family

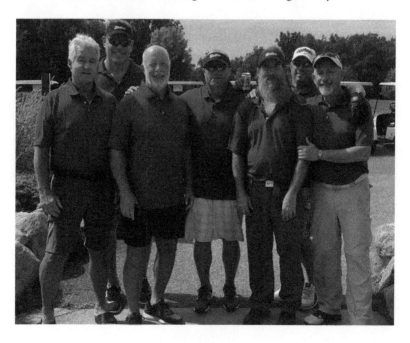

Annual Dirtbag –sons/son-in-law with Tom, Greg & Pat

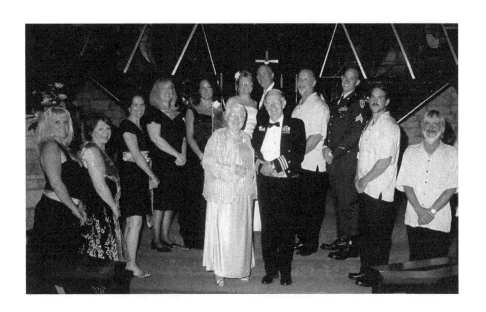

A Great Wedding Day

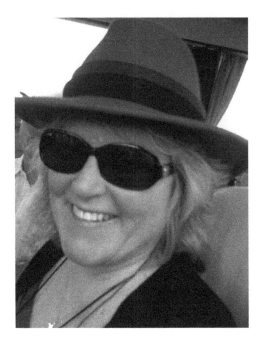

MK's fave hat

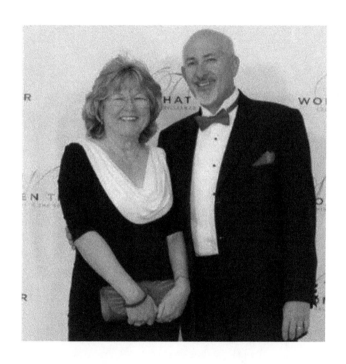

One of our dressiest pictures

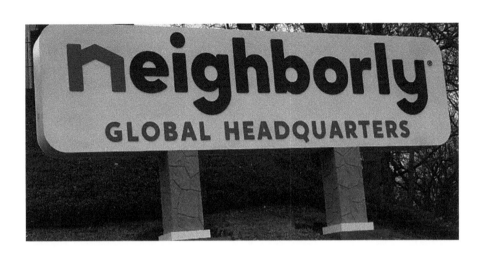

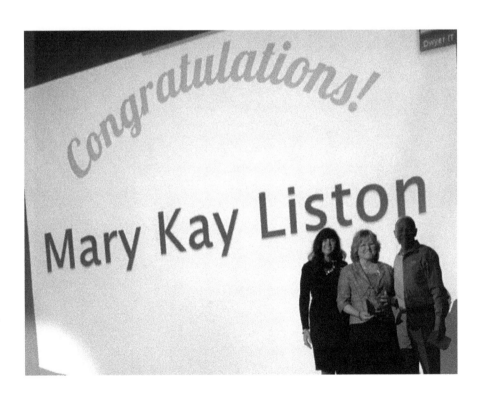

Work home for 10 years where MK won numerous awards with COO Mary and CEO Mike

Diagnosed

Section 11: 76 Days

Thursday, November 3, 2022

Day 1

A week or two before I had woken up in the middle of the night with sharp pains on the right side of my chest. Shortly thereafter I developed a nasty cough—but not the kind that brings anything up. Each cough made it feel like there was a knife going into the upper portion of my chest.

A week later I got the same pain on the left side— now it was on both sides. The cough persisted and along with the cough came this horrendous smell—to the point of needing breath mints. Slowly the pain on the right side subsided and the pain on the left side lessened.

Mary Kay talked to her sister, Micki, one night. Mick is a nurse practitioner. She recommended MK take me to urgent care the next day. At this point we were still in our Ohio summer home and urgent care was less than a mile away.

Immediately they did a cardiogram and took blood. The cardiogram was fine, which was a relief for me. Dad died of a heart attack at 54, my brother died of a heart attack at 61, and my son, Andy, now forty-five, had 99% blockage in two places in his widow maker at 38, which resulted in a double bypass.

The doctor came in and said there were three things he was very worried about and recommended I get to the ER—by ambulance—immediately. This shocked us because I could've walked to the ER in less time than it would take for an ambulance to pick me up and take me over.

The next four hours were spent in the ER. The chest X-ray was the first screening. It showed that I had two masses in my right lung.

Then came more blood tests, a cardiogram, and finally a CT scan with contrast dye.

About 45 minutes later, the ER doctor came in with a somber look on his face and announced that he was sorry to tell us that it looked like lung cancer. He said we need to get an oncologist right away.

Our life had changed with the words "It looks like you have lung cancer."

Here I am. 68 years old. Three kids. I think I'm healthy. Been an asthmatic but an Albuterol rescue inhaler, one cartridge per month, handles everything.

We had both been looking forward to retirement for years. Finally, all those years of working and not living by the kids because of our jobs had paid off and we are set! We are snowbirds with a house about thirty miles outside of Cleveland within ten miles of Andy and Sarah, our son and daughter-in-law, and their two boys, Noah, and Isaiah. Our other son, Marcus, and five of his kids are also close – with his oldest, Tyler, now stationed at the Air Force base in Great Falls, MT.

In the past couple of years, both Mary Kay and I had squamous cell skin cancer that our dermatologist cut out. We never treated that as "real" cancer.

I've never smoked. I've never worked in an environment that could cause this. My dad smoked until he died in 1967— so I hadn't been around significant secondhand smoke for over 50 years. As the doctor left, MK and I hugged, cried, then prayed and gave it to God.

That night we called the three kids. We were scheduled to spend the winter months in Florida, just two miles down the road from our daughter Jae and her husband, Jeff. We told them that we weren't sure if we would seek treatment in Ohio or head to Florida and do it there—just six weeks earlier than planned.

We immediately sent a note to our primary care physician in Florida and let her know we needed to talk to her ASAP. A call was scheduled for the next morning at 10.

Friday, November 4, 2022

Day 2

By 9:30 the next morning, daughter, Jae, had already set an appointment for me with her pulmonologist for the 10th—which was also MK's birthday. Happy birthday, honey. Jae, like me, was a lifelong asthmatic and had worked with Dr. K for years. She knew I'd be well cared for by him.

We love our primary care physician, Trish. She is also Jae's PCP and Jae told us she was fabulous. The first words out of Trish's mouth when we told her what had happened the day before were "Oh shit!"

She went on to tell us to get our butts to Florida as soon as possible, so that I didn't need to be breathing that frigid winter air of Ohio. (We hadn't thought of that). She also knew Dr. K and had collaborated with him at one of the hospitals. "He is awesome— he and I will take care of all of this for you."

By noon we had our flights to Florida four days away.

Saturday, November 5 -
Wednesday November 9

Days 3-7

It was time to line up the prayer warriors. I had heard the term used in other situations but never in our lives. We didn't want it announced on Facebook, so we were careful who we told.

Pastor Marissa, of Good Soil Lutheran in Rocky River, Ohio, is our pastor and we wanted her to be involved right away. Then we contacted a select few friends and the rest of the family. Just a couple of criteria: they wouldn't put it on Facebook, and they would pray for us.

The first people we thought about as prayer warriors were Douglas and Elizabeth Rogers. Not only are they great friends, but Doug was responsible for so much of Mary Kay's corporate success.

We know that the hand of God brought Mary Kay to the VP position at Mr. Appliance. Doug was the president of the company and over our time together they became close friends.

Doug gave so much more to people than he ever asked. No surprise when they suggested that they Facetime us each Monday night to learn the latest and offer a prayer. What great Christian friends! You read Doug's story earlier in this book.

Thursday, November 10, 2022

Day 8

Happy 68th birthday to MK! This amazing Christian woman has been such a blessing in my life for the last 20 years. She is my best friend. We love spending time together.

Researchers estimate that 41% of all first marriages end in divorce. Sixty percent of second marriages also end in divorce. Here ends the myth—we live and learn. I get it. I'm part of this state. Why? I got married to Joan when we were both eighteen and had three kids by the time, we were twenty-two. How prepared do you think we were for either? Heck, I was still a boy who just acted like a man and didn't take anyone's advice. I surely wasn't going to listen to my mother in this area and my dad had already died so I was left to my own devices.

I can confidently say that Mary Kay and I have never had a fight. That isn't to say we haven't disagreed on things, but nothing is worth fighting about. We've never gone to bed mad at each other. Why should we?

We met Jae at Dr. K's office. Jae said that she noticed that my breathing sounded terrible when she and her husband, Jeff, were up in Ohio staying with us over Halloween weekend.

Dr. K wasn't sure what the problem was but wanted to make sure we got the biopsy done as soon as possible. He gave me the COPD test and found that my lung capacity was at 50%. Not good; not horrid. Jae was right: I didn't sound like I should've.

Dr. K told us that once the biopsy was done it would take about two weeks to see whether it was cancer.

He also showed us, based on the CT scan from Ohio, that the mass was close to my chest cavity, making a biopsy easy to do.

Weekend - November 11-13

Days 9-11

So hard to learn patience. I was NEVER a patient person in my life. I am a Type A personality who tries to make things happen – not let things happen.

"Thy Will Be Done" to me was more of a "Thy Will Be Done—but I have a few suggestions along the way, Lord." He obviously doesn't need my help. He knows, fortunately, that I need His. And left to my own devices— well, He knows my history!

Monday, November 14

Day 12

A person's mind sure can run away with negative thoughts, can't it? Dr. K let me know that the biopsy was now approved, and the hospital would let me know when they could do it. I thought this was going to be an immediate thing.

I've always enjoyed great writers, especially those who have a wonderful sense of humor, tell exceptional stories, and make me want to keep reading and finish the book or article. Terry Pluto is one of the greats.

We have been reading Terry's book, *Faith and You – Volume 1* during our morning devotions. Terry is a great faith writer, also an outstanding sportswriter at the Cleveland Plain Dealer. I'd heard about him but didn't really get acquainted with him until I found his weekly column in the *Sunday Plain Dealer*, "Faith and You."

We read a chapter titled "Why is it so hard to pray out loud?" What I loved about this chapter is that it's so easy for us to say, "I'll pray for you," but few people ever say, "Can I pray WITH you right now?" What a wonderful lesson.

This is why I like having Pastor Marissa or Doug and Liz pray with us. It is always aloud, and they don't do "King James Version prayers" with thee's and thou's. They talk to God like they are talking to their best friend. I know why: because God is their best friend!

Tuesday, November 15
Day 13

I got a call from the hospital— biopsy was set for 1 p.m. November 29. Time to let a few people know.

First, I called three guys I refer to as closest buddies to share the latest. David, Greg, and Chris.

I went to junior high and all high school with David. We lived less than a mile apart then and would double-date often. Both of us had a midnight curfew. I remember like it was yesterday dropping David off at 11:58, then flying home to pull in the driveway by midnight.

Greg attended the same junior high, just two years behind us. I had just come from a parochial school with thirty-five kids, max, in a class. Now here I was with hundreds of kids in a class. What shocked me the most was the swimming class. We still talk about it. The boys swam naked in swimming class. Really!

I knew Greg in high school, too, but I didn't find out who he really was until I was about twenty. We played softball together, some hoops, and lots of golf. For years I had asked to buy his putter because I had one round with him where I hit only ten putts in nine holes. I'm not that good at golf; I knew it had to be the putter.

We played one more time before I moved to Florida in 2002. When we were done Greg said he had a going-away present for me. It was his putter—the one I still play with today. Of course, we both cried and hugged that day before I drove away.

I met Chris at work in Ohio in 1981. I remember walking into Kinetico, a water treatment manufacturer in Newbury, Ohio, for the first time and looking around for someone I thought I could spend time together with. Joan and the kids were still in Illinois and would be for some time. Chris and I met and that was it.

On the drive to find a place I had rented from an ad in the paper, I was stuck in a snowstorm on I-90, along with everyone else on I-90 that day, for over an hour. I had a bed, a TV, pots and pans, and new wingtips in the car.

The next day I woke up at 5:30 a.m., all excited for the new job. I went out to leave in plenty of time but had to hitchhike the ten miles to work because my car wouldn't start in the 35-below weather. Luckily, I only needed two rides.

Chris and I were the same age, but our backgrounds were vastly different. He was a brilliant engineer. I didn't understand what he was drawing even after he explained it to me.

There are only about four hundred stories about the two of us after that. Most good. All funny. When Joan and I split before our divorce I moved into Chris's. Took a waterbed that we put on the landing upstairs between two bedrooms, a desk, and some clothes. He got me through life in the first year after the divorce. It was a trip to Florida together in his Trans Am with T-Top where we had double dates waiting for us. Those dates didn't work out.

However, we did stop by this campsite to see a girl I knew from the racquet ball club I worked at after I finished my day job so I could afford to pay for the kids to go there, too. She was staying with her parents. I wanted to date her – but was just getting to know her. She and Chris connected immediately, and now Chris and Gay are going on 40 years of marriage. MK and I just love hanging out with them as much as we can.

David now lives back in Rockford where we both grew up, Chris in Ohio – about twelve miles from our house up North. Greg lives within ten miles of us in Florida. Three guys that I can call at 3 a.m. and tell them I need them now and know that they'll leave in the next 20 minutes or so. People like that I call real friends.

"You're the average of the five people you spend the most time with."

I wish I could take credit for this gem. I can't. Motivational speaker Jim Rohn said this. Was he ever right!

I don't mind if anyone ever compares me to Chris, David, or Greg. We are all quite different, but our hearts are the same. Our relationship with people is the same. And we truly do love each other as brothers.

Monday, November 21, 2022

Day 19

This was the night for Doug and Liz's call with us. I have so many wonderful memories with them. Doug became part of our men's group at church on Wednesday mornings. For Doug to get to a 6:30 a.m. meeting meant waking up before 4 a.m. to get his body ready.

When we see people who are disabled, we often have no idea what they go through to live a "normal" life. I've traveled with Doug—including on his first trip without Liz. Doug is always the first one on an airplane and the last one to get off. There is a special wheelchair that fits between the aisle seats. Getting an Uber is also different. We had to get one that could carry a wheelchair.

Doug has managed his issues over the past eight years better than most people manage a sprain. He also goes out of his way to help people who might be feeling sorry for themselves.

I volunteered years ago to be on the Prayer Team at our church in Cleveland, Good Soil Lutheran. So, every week I get a list of all the people the church was praying for, and then MK and I pray for them daily. On this day, I saw my name on the list with the comment: "Undergoing test this month to determine a potential cancer diagnosis."

Tuesday, November 22, 2022

Day 20

Jae's 49th birthday. I couldn't be old enough to have a child who was entering her 50th year of life. She was a blessing at 7 a.m. on Thanksgiving morning 49 years ago and she is such a blessing today.

Long ago, I started a tradition that I plan to continue my whole life. My goal is to be the first one to wish my kids Happy Birthday. I'll set my alarm to wake me up at 11:58pm so I can text them "Happy Birthday" just as the clock hits midnight. Years ago, I simply called them. But as they got older, texting became more important than phone calls to all three of them, so by now it's a text. Plus, the text message has a time stamp letting them know when I texted.

We have a couple of family members who are raising other people's kids. I'm so glad they are—but think about this:

I can think of a handful of great parents out there. I mean great at building boys into men, girls into women, all kids into contributing members of society who have a magnificent work ethic. College kids who are more interested in graduating in four years with a degree versus spending however long it takes because Mom and Dad are paying for it anyway and don't ever want to miss a fun time!

I had great parents. Everything I've accomplished in life was because of their guidance. They told me "No" when other parents were trying to be their kid's best friend. I learned by watching them. Listening to them. Seeing how they interacted with people. I learned their ethics by simply observing them.

I am confident that my three kids will tell you that I am a much better father today than I was when they were little. I listen better. I have way more patience. I spend quality time with them. I'm glad that God that gave me the opportunity to become a much better father and that I've been able to help others be the best parents they can be.

Wednesday, November 23, 2022

Day 21

I got an email from a hospital last night asking if I knew what the leading cause of cancer deaths was last year. Yep. LUNG CANCER. Accounted for 23% of all cancer deaths. In 2020, 63,135 females and 72,949 males.

I never smoked—anything—and now I was waiting for a biopsy to see if I had it.

"Thy will be done."

Thursday, November 24, 2022
- Thanksgiving

Day 22

Thanksgiving wishes this early morning as I sat in my office at the computer and MK was still asleep.

I wish MK could have met my dad at Pepsi. I loved going to Dad's work after school. The bus would drop me off in front of the plant and I'd stay there with Dad until he went home.

I remember vividly sitting a wooden 24-bottle carrier on its end for my chair, then pulling up to his desk to do my homework on the metal pull-out shelf. He always gave me two nickels: one for pop and one for a candy bar.

It was at work where I got one of the major lessons of my life. My brother, Duke, worked for Pepsi as a route driver. He was training a new guy, John, one day. At the end of the day Duke said he wanted to introduce John to our dad. He said, "John, this is my old man; Dad this is John."

With that, Dad looked sternly at him and said, "Duke, don't ever call me your old man again I'm your dad or your father." Then he walked back to his office.

After that day I never called any person "old man," and I never heard my brother do it either. It was all about respect.

Dad taught me the value of credit. I still remember the lesson even though I was in the third grade. Duke needed to buy a car and asked Dad to cosign it for him. Dad told me, "Your brother doesn't pay his bills on time and the bank doesn't trust him to pay them back. I'm cosigning because we have good credit, and they know that I will pay them back if he doesn't. I've never been late on any payments in my life."

The words that still burn in my mind are "Your word is your bond." Another great lesson from Dad.

On the bottom shelf of our refrigerator was a six pack of special export beer in case a guest wanted a drink. I never saw Dad drink even one can.

Instead, he'd have a bowl of ice cream every night and tell me that he saved his beer money for ice cream.

Lessons galore and I don't remember him ever "preaching to me." Didn't have to.

The night he died changed my life forever. I was in eighth grade. He had a heart attack at 54. Died instantly. I'm sure the two packs of Camel unfiltered cigarettes every day since he was in high school were contributing factors. On the way to the hospital, I remember praying the 23rd Psalm. All the years at St. Paul, where I went to grade school since kindergarten, gave me a wonderful upbringing on the Bible and in trusting God. I missed the lessons and guidance he would have given me in those formative high school years. I missed having my dad see my kids.

To survive, Mom got a job for the first time since Duke had been born. We lived half a mile from the hospital, and we took in nursing students to help pay the bills. We purchased the house just six months before Dad died. All we had was $10,000 in life insurance—not enough to come close to paying for the house. Mom had never balanced the checkbook and suddenly everything changed in her life.

After he died, I found a letter Dad had written but never sent to his father-in-law. It was dated January 12, 1942. I believe my mom was having a nervous breakdown and he sent her back home to be with her parents so they could help with Duke, seven at the time, and get my mom to eat properly. He put them on a train to Pinckneyville, Illinois- about 315 miles south of Chicago and a small town.

One of the excerpts is as follows:

Pop, I sure hope Alyne [my mom] is feeling just fine again. She sure was feeling bad and I didn't know what to do for her. I'm glad to hear that you are making her eat. Good, boy I couldn't. I think that will help a lot along with a lot of good rest.

Pop, I hope you don't mind if I ask you for some advice – but I sure would like to find out what your opinion is. I think Alyne, Dukie and I would be a lot better off getting away from this

big city [Chicago]. If I got home at regular times each day, we could all eat together. I know Alyne would eat better.
[The challenge is that] I'm in a secure job and have been with this company for six ½ years. I started at $15 per week and now I make $37.50 per week. But I know as soon as things start going downhill again my pay will slide down the rest of it. We have no wage or hour law in our company as far as my job is concerned. Boy, I sure would like to know what you think. [Remember, this was in the middle of World War II]
Well, Pop, I'll be looking forward to your answer. Give my best wishes to everyone. With love, your son, Ted.

I thought it was strange that I found this specific letter. Eventually, I found out why he didn't send it. My grandfather died that day—January 12, 1942. Dad must have written this then got a phone call or a telegram.

What touched me was that, at 29 years old, he was asking his father-in-law for advice. Plus, he signed the letter "your son."

I thought about how blessed I was. To grow up in a house with a dad like that. A Dad who had a Bible in his desk and when one of his employees had an issue he would bring them into his office, shut the door, and try and counsel them based on Biblical principles.

I remember when this happened to Jerry. His brother, Leon, was killed in a car accident and Jerry was having a tough time getting through it. Dad brought him into his office and opened the Bible to find what the Lord said about this situation. Wow–what a man of God.

Today is Thanksgiving. So many things to be thankful for.

I'm so blessed to have great friends who are now prayer warriors. To have been blessed with wonderful pastors at the various churches we've attended with our many moves.

To be in Florida, just two miles from Jae, with 78-degree weather in November—and no snow!

I'm so blessed. Just a little inconvenient right now.

Friday, November 25, 2022 –
Day after Thanksgiving

Day 23

It was a quiet day yesterday early morning. Jae and Jeff had travelled to Ohio for a Thanksgiving weekend with her brother and her mom. We didn't have any plans and we had plenty of leftovers from our early Thanksgiving dinner with Jae and Jeff earlier in the week.

The call came from Marti, MK's sister, just two years younger than MK. She was in the hospital again in Orlando. Her health issues started five years ago with breast cancer. More recently she had repeated issues with tumors on her pancreas. Fortunately, they were non-cancerous, but they kept coming back, necessitating more surgeries.

She spoke to MK for a minute and then asked to talk to me. Usually her conversations are with MK, so it seemed odd.

She told me that the pulmonologist came into her room this morning announcing that she had a mass in her lungs, and they thought it might be lung cancer. Sounded like what happened 23 days ago to me. She wanted me to break the news to MK.

Based on my conversation, MK understood what was happening. We were the only ones who knew—they hadn't told their kids yet. MK asked Marti if we could come to the hospital right away and visit.

The drive to the hospital took less than two hours, and we had a wonderful unplanned day with them once we arrived. We could easily relate to her latest news.

On our way home after the visit MK and I discussed how blessed we were to be able to join them for the day. If I had gotten the prognosis, I had we would have still been in Ohio.

God works in mysterious ways. "Thy will be done."

Saturday, November 26, 2022
Day 24

My early mornings when MK was still sleeping were the time when my mind was just racing. Today it was about what would happen three days from now during the biopsy.

I didn't know how long the biopsy itself would take. The hospital told me to plan on being there for two to four hours after the biopsy to make sure the lung didn't collapse. That doesn't happen often but if it did, they would just have admitted me for one night, most likely.

It is good that doctors are honest today. They don't say, "Stay a few hours just to make sure all went well with the biopsy"! Now they say, "in case your lung collapses!" I preferred the old way.

The irony is that I felt great!

Sunday, November 27, 2022
Day 25

Went back to my "dad" file and it brought back more memories. Dad's best friend, Lyle, had been asking him for years to leave Pepsi and become the plant manager of his company. Lyle's son was my best friend at St. Paul. Dad didn't want to join Lyle just because they were friends. He wanted to be sure it was the right thing to do.

I found a letter Dad wrote to the owners of the Pepsi franchise after a promotion, and he was considering leaving. These are a few excerpts:

> *In recent years, my attitude has changed toward my approach to everyday living. Some things that used to seem important to*

me are now of very little importance. Other values are growing in me, and some have even matured. I will only attempt to cover items that affect the subject matter at hand so that you will better understand me.

I begin by saying that I have come to realize as never before that I have a father in heaven and that his son, Jesus Christ, died a horrible death in my place for my sins. Recognizing that I am still sinful and this I know by seeing my reflection in the mirror and the ten Commandments, I have a real need for a Savior. Therefore, my intentions are to serve my Lord in any way that I can – my first obligation is to him – my first obligation is to him because without him I would have no assurance of eternal life.

I will in no way let this affect my work and will continue to perform to the best of my ability as long as I am in your employ.

Now don't misunderstand this – I still have an obligation to my family and expect to support them to the best of the ability God has given me.

To you, my employer, I also have some obligation. You also have an obligation to me the employee and since I am sure you would bring it to your attention if I did not fulfill my obligation to you, and rightfully so, I am bringing the matter to your attention. [This was regarding compensation when he was promoted but received no financial changes in pay.]

Please don't read between the lines because I just don't write, talk, or do business with hidden meanings.

Quite frankly, I have prayed over this matter, asking for guidance. Recognizing that I am more emotional than some people, I was afraid that if I spoke to you about this, I might not express myself right and might misunderstand. Please forgive me if I have offended you.

He did leave. This is the person I was always proud to call Dad. It was amazing how he molded me in the first 13 years of my life. I never had one sad day with Dad—ever. Not one bad memory. I am blessed.

I loved going to church with Dad. I couldn't wait until Dad, and I could usher together. I also hoped Duke would be part of our same usher team.

I ushered today, MK helped serve communion. But it was different with Dad.

Pastor Rita retired recently. She was our pastor in Florida. The irony is that she is the mother of Pastor Marissa, our pastor in Ohio. In the Lutheran church we first hire interim pastors for 12 to 15 months before we find the permanent pastor. I didn't think MK and I would last those 12 months without church shopping. It was just too different without Pastor R's love.

Monday, November 28, 2022
Day 26

Today we had an appointment with a Florida attorney to update our wills and related documents. We wanted to make changes from what we had planned in Texas. So glad we did. Age = wisdom. If anything should happen to me now or 20 years from now I don't want MK to suddenly become the wicked stepmother. Jae is the administrator for our will and knows where everything is in our house regarding this.

A Wisconsin friend of mine sold mausoleum spaces. He told me about the sale he couldn't make. When the husband went to the bathroom, the wife whispered to him that her husband had stage 4 cancer and didn't want to face it. He died less than a month later leaving nothing taken care of for his wife.

It is important to make your wishes known if you have young children, too. I always wanted to choose who would have my kids—not leave that decision to the state. I don't care if you're 30 or 60—take care of it.MK and I are big believers that one needs to have everything set for their kids—regardless of the parents' age. And, if married, have things prepared for their spouse. I've been a believer in this since my grandma died when I was just a kid, and my dad was alive.

Grandma Liston had already met at the funeral home and had her arrangements all done and paid for. This included the dress she would wear, the flag she wanted on the coffin, the coffin picked out and paid for— everything. When she died my dad and uncle, both of her sons, went to the funeral home and just signed the papers she had already taken care of. Easy.

When Dad died in 1967 it was not only shocking, but nothing was ready! Mom didn't really understand the financial stuff. We went to the same funeral home that my grandma had used but nothing was prepared in advance. Stress on everyone.

One of the things that will happen to you if you are going through a health scare like his one, or any other one with medical issues, is that you might miss things that are particularly important to you.

A case in point is our son-in-law's birthday on the 26th. Already sent his card but I made a big deal, personally, of that midnight text. He didn't get one this year. Got to remember next year!

Tuesday, November 29, 2022
Day 27

Biopsy day. The procedure was at 1 p.m. but we needed to be there at 11. Jae picked us up as the hospital is just a mile or so from Jae's. She sat with MK for the afternoon while I went in and then waited, after the biopsy, to see if my lungs collapsed or not.

Not worried at all. This has been the next step for me in the process of who knows how many processes lie ahead. Perspective makes it easier to keep my eye on smaller targets.

It helps to break it down into small steps:

- Process of finding the right doctor
- Process of choosing the hospital for the biopsy
- Process of finding out about the biopsy
- Process of what to do after we found out the results

For now, we are waiting for the results.

Doug and Liz's prayer session was wonderful last night. Got lots of love from my boys last night, too. Great devotions with MK this morning.

OK, Lord, it is in your hands. And I'm really trying hard to remember, "Thy will be done."

Wednesday, November 30, 2022
Day 28

Reflections on the day yesterday.

The biopsy was easy. No pain. Got an IV portal where medicines could be injected to numb the chest. They warned me it might cause what would feel like a super brain freeze. Crickets. Nothing. No discomfort whatsoever.

Doctors did have to come back one time because they needed more tissue for the biopsy.

The mass is about the size of a Ping-Pong ball. Another mass, too, that is much smaller, but they didn't need to biopsy that one.

I'm a hairy guy so I shaved my chest, just in case. Nothing like tape being pulled off a hairy arm or hairy chest. I now looked like a 12-year-old boy with white hair.

Lori, the surgical nurse, came in and said she needed to clean up the back of my arm. She has been with Trinity Hospital, where I got the biopsy, for 30 years. I noticed some red stuff on the back of my gown. Yep, a bunch of blood. So, she changed the gown, put on the bandage, and I was good as new.

Now, wait. Up to two weeks.

Thursday, December 1, 2022
Day 29: The Scare

First thoughts today were for my brother, Duke. He would have been 87 today. It's been 26 years since he died. My parents were forty when I was born, and Duke was almost nineteen and in college. He and I never lived in the same house.

On May 10, 1997, I got a call from my nephew in Las Cruces where the entire family lived. He told me that my brother had died. Whew. Sixty-one years old. That was a tough one. We weren't close but weren't NOT close, either. When I graduated from high school, he got me a job in the factory where he worked. I worked 3rd shift and made the decision then that I'd never work in a factory again in my life. I never did. Not that it was beneath me—it was just so physically hard!

On the one hand, that decision worked out well. On the other hand, I would never finish college.

Dr. K called me today and said they got preliminary results from the biopsy. Looks now like it is *not* lung cancer. He thinks, however, it is lymphoma—which is still cancer. (How'd you like the play, Mrs. Lincoln?) He also wants me to get an oncologist right away. He mentioned there were some inconsistencies, and they sent the biopsy to the University of Michigan for their specialists to review.

I didn't understand this because I thought we would want the results before we called in an oncologist.

MK called Dr. Trish (our PCP) right away. Dr. Trish asked if Dr. K thought it was Hodgkin's or non-Hodgkin's. Of course, we had no idea the answer, even if Dr. K might have mentioned it. She sent us the names of a couple of oncologists at Moffitt Cancer Center in Tampa. We put those names in our pocket.

The best part of the day, however, was receiving a card from Pastor Marissa. Inside were the words, "I can do all things through Christ who strengthens me. Philippians 4:13." Just another reason we love our pastor and believe attending the church with a pastor who genuinely cares about you is so important.

Tonight, I prayed for patience as it was going to take another week or two before we would get the final word on the biopsy from U of M.

Friday, December 2, 2022
Day 30

I love the attitude of Dr. Trish. Thursday was such a scary day! She told us today that it might not be lymphoma. It might just be a severe strain of pneumonia. She explained that it is a good thing that they sent the biopsy to U of M and the specialists there.

I called Gay, my lifelong friend Chris's wife, and asked her not to share with Chris yet that we are looking at lymphoma. He is having an exceedingly challenging time with all of this. He was afraid, she said, that the last time we saw them in Ohio would be the last time. What a great brother.

Saturday, December 3, 2022

Day 31

Lots of time to think about life these days. Many times, my mind goes back to my dad and all the lessons I learned from him. Watching how my boys are, how they are like dads, how they are as husbands or mates, reminds me of me in so many ways. This isn't necessarily good. I wish I'd had the wisdom as a young father that I do as "young grandfather."

My dad never gave me a bad lesson in life. If anything, my mom complained that he worked too hard and too many hours. But I never felt short-changed by his time.

My parents got involved with school and church. Must be a Liston thing. Mom on the PTA and doing a bunch of committees and Dad ushering every Sunday at the 7 a.m. service. He was the first one there every Sunday and made sure he welcomed everyone at the door. No one had done this before. Mom complained that he should be sleeping in one day a week, but his priority was being at the first service on Sunday mornings.

We were the Nelsons or the Cleavers. Dad worked, Mom stayed home to help raise me, Dad came home for lunch every day and home for dinner every night. I was raised like an only child.

Dad was involved with the school board at St. Paul, and he helped organize the first class at Rockford Lutheran high school. I found the speech that he wrote for eighth grade graduation at St. Paul in 1964. Excerpts are:

> *The Bible says "wisdom is the principal thing, therefore get wisdom and in all getting, get understanding" – Proverbs 4:7. The test of your understanding is yet to come. In this direction I refer you to the epistle of James Chapter 1, verse twenty-two, which says, "Be ye doers of the word and not hearers only, deceiving your own selves." In other words, it is not enough to remember what we hear and be able to repeat it, write it or*

*preserve what we have written – we must be doers of the words,
or we are only fooling ourselves.
This is your final test – the result of which will also be graded
but this time by the greatest teacher this world has ever known
– our Lord and Savior Jesus Christ.
May God go with each of you and through God's grace may you
receive the gift of wisdom, understanding and courage to face
this world unafraid and unashamed to be doers of the word.
To the end, that others will come to learn of our blessed Savior.*

My mom carried little Gideon Bibles in her purse. We didn't live in a great area of town. One night, when Dad was working late, we got home after dark and started to go into the house. Mom was a terrible "car parker" and needed to move the car much closer to the curb. I stayed on the porch with my schoolbook bag and her purse. We lived on a corner, and I noticed someone had crossed the street and walked down the sidewalk next to the house. Suddenly the man walked onto the porch, picked up my bag and my mom's purse and hurried away.

I wonder what he thought when he didn't find any money in the purse and discovered a dozen little Gideon Bibles?

I liked how I was raised. No computers. No cell phones. Only three stations on the TV that you had to get up and change yourself. Having to hang wash on a clothesline outside. Finding kids in the neighborhood to play football, baseball, and basketball with. Of course, Dad put the basketball hoop up on our garage.

I know that I have lived an outstanding life. So glad, however, that MK is here with me as we face this together.

Sunday, December 4, 2022
Day 32

Family. It's such a blessing. I look at MK's remaining family of five sisters. Their brother died eighteen months ago of ALS. It's such a nasty disease. More than seventeen million people took the "Ice Bucket Challenge" for ALS a few years ago. The stunt raised over $2.5 million. Pray for those people who have ALS.

MK and I talked again tonight about how our lives were so different when we were growing up. I was in one grade school, one junior high and one high school. MK changed schools every two years. My dad was home every night. MK's dad was gone up to six months at a time—twelve months when he went to Vietnam.

Monday, December 5, 2022
Day 33

The roller coaster.

Dr. K called; could the biopsy results be back? Yes . . . not so fast, Skippy.

We spoke with Dr. K's nurse. She said to come by the office and pick up the paperwork. She told us we needed to contact Moffitt Cancer Center. They were the best around and one of the best in the country. They often recommend a different oncologist based on the type of cancer a patient has—let's say lung cancer vs. lymphoma.

MK called Moffitt and found those that Dr. Trish had recommended couldn't get me in quickly, but Dr. C could get me in at 7:50 a.m. next Tuesday. *Great*—I think. We called Greg's daughter-in-law, Heidi, who worked at Moffitt as a nurse practitioner. She knew the doctor well and said he was great, and we would love him.

We finished our day with prayer warriors Doug and Liz. He sure was uplifting!

It is especially important for people facing cancer or any other scary illness to surround themselves with the right kind of people. People who aren't telling you what to do; those who love you . . . and *like* you! People who will pray with you aloud.

Tuesday, December 6, 2022

Day 34

I'm tired most days during the day and need, or at least want, a nap. I'm not sure if it is physical or emotional or if I'm just getting older. It certainly can't be that!

The process is mentally and emotionally wearing me out. Dr. K's call yesterday reminded me that there is a biopsy that will, no doubt, decide what I can or can't do for the upcoming months. We have trips planned that I really want to go on, but we are in limbo now. For an impatient person like me, waiting is difficult.

All the Christmas decorations are in tubs, waiting for us to dive in and make the house look quite different. I brought them in from the garage on Sunday.

As we were returning to Florida last year from Ohio on December 21 we dreaded all the decorating we had to do so quickly. Driving up to our house, we were shocked! Jae and her thirty-year-old stepdaughter had already made the house look beautiful. Lights on the bushes. A wreath she found in our attic that we didn't know we had. Cabinets decorated. A bunch of new stuff that Jae ordered. She told us that it was our Christmas present—and it was impressive.

We were both concerned that we wouldn't be able to duplicate her efforts, so we took pictures of everything last year to remind us.

I have to say we did a decent job.

Working that hard putting up decorations might earn me a nap today!

Wednesday, December 7, 2022
Day 35

Decorating the house yesterday for Christmas did a surprisingly excellent job of taking my mind off the biopsy results. Of course, I'm anxious, but it hasn't been two weeks yet.

Looking at the beautiful Christmas tree reminds me of when I was a kid with asthma. My mom went overboard to make sure we didn't have any dust in the house that might aggravate it. I'm sure it drove my dad crazy. At Christmas, the tree was the worst.

Have you ever seen those silver trees made of aluminum branches? You know they looked like aluminum foil. Along with those trees came a "wheel" of red, green, yellow, and blue that turned, giving the tree those colors. As a kid I wanted a real tree. As an adult I had one, traipsing through the snow up North to cut one down. Shades of "Christmas Vacation." I was Clark Griswold eyeing the right size tree for our living room. I'm over that, and the artificial tree we have is fine.

Thursday, December 8, 2022

Day 36

I wake up every morning hoping that Dr. K will call with the biopsy results. How long ago was November 29th when I got the biopsy? Nine months? Ten years? I felt like it was. Although I pray daily for patience, I admit I don't have very much of it.

Dr. K has prescribed sodium tablets because my sodium levels were low. Those of us who played football on teams when we were kids remember taking sodium tablets to prevent overheating. But today I couldn't find them at any drug store, health food store or anywhere else. Finally, I found a pharmacy that would order them. I'm hopeful they will raise my levels before my next blood test.

Marcus's oldest son, Tyler, turned 23today. He joined the Air Force two and a half years ago and is stationed at Malmstrom AFB in Montana. Not sure if he will be a lifer or not.

We certainly enjoy a patriotic thread throughout our family.

Marcus is just finishing his 20th year in the Army. Three tours of duty as a combat medic and several years in the National Guard. It was on one of his returns home that I noticed that he had post-traumatic stress disorder (PTSD) symptoms: when we went to a restaurant, he made sure nothing was behind him and he had to face the door. When he drove, he wouldn't drive in the right-hand lane – that is where the roadside bombs were planted.

MK's Dad was career Navy. Her family lived at a secret Navy base on the West Coast. If you've seen the movie "The Hunt for Red October" you have seen how Navy ships laid cable at the bottom of the ocean so they could listen for submarine activity from our enemies. That is what this command did.

Years before, it was her dad's 40th birthday, the day the USS Pueblo was captured. Here is how the History Channel describes it:

*On January 23, 1968, the USS Pueblo, a Navy intelligence
vessel, is engaged in routine surveillance of the North Korean
coast when it is intercepted by North Korean patrol boats.
According to U.S. reports, the Pueblo was in international
waters almost sixteen miles from shore, but the North Koreans
turned their guns on the lightly armed vessel and demanded
its surrender. The Americans attempted to escape, and the
North Koreans opened fire, wounding the commander and
two others. With capture inevitable, the Americans stalled
for time, destroying the classified information aboard while
taking further fire. Several more crew members were wounded.*

MK's family was stationed in Japan then. Dad got a call, said he had
to go, and was gone for two weeks. He oversaw communications between
the Pacific Fleet and Washington, D.C., and played a key role in managing
the crisis.

MK laughs about when Dad retired after 27 years. Immediately he
became a Junior ROTC instructor at a high school in Las Vegas. He got to
wear his uniform khakis. His entire work life he never had to learn how to
dress like the rest of us.

Friday, December 9, 2022
Day 37

Tonight, we will see For King and Country in Tampa. Since our introduc-
tion to Casting Crowns, we have attended concerts by Christian music
groups and our car radios are typically tuned to Christian music.

Our first concert with Doug and Liz introduced us to Compassion
International and sponsoring kids overseas for only $38 per month. We
have volunteered at Compassion events since then, and this was one of them.

We were supposed to see the "Little Drummer Boy" concert in Cleveland with son, Marcus, and his date before coming down to Florida, but our hurried change of schedule made us miss that one. Marcus went, though, and really enjoyed it. When we saw that the group was coming to Tampa, we immediately got tickets. I'm excited for tonight!

Saturday, December 10, 2022

Day 38

Woke up thinking about heading to Moffitt Cancer Center on Monday morning. There is something unsettling about going to a cancer center— even if it is only to talk to a doctor.

To me it says, "You've got cancer." I don't want to be the first in my family to die of cancer. Of course, we were quick to die of heart attacks, but no one has had the big C word.

Sunday, December 11, 2022

Day 39

Two weeks until Christmas. Three weeks until New Years. Yet, no biopsy results. (How am I doing on this thing called "patience"?)

We've been missing our retired pastor, Pastor Rita. Glad she could retire but going to church hasn't been the same. I'm thinking we might need to go church shopping sooner than later, even though MK and I are both involved in the service. It just isn't the same.

Thinking about our trip to the cancer center tomorrow. Hoping it isn't a waste of time for them or for us without the biopsy results.

Monday, December 12, 2022

Day 40

There is something weird about going to a renowned cancer center when you don't know if you have cancer or not—but are quite sure you do based on what the doctors have said and seen so far.

All we heard about Moffitt Cancer Center in Tampa is that it is one of the best. When it comes to health issues, that is exactly where I want to be – at one of the best. It has been two weeks since the biopsy on the 29th of November. Seems like a year.

Reminds me when I was looking for a job because I got downsized. You stare at your phone praying it will ring with good news. It has happened to me a couple of times, so I understand what a challenging time that is in a person's life.

Thinking you have cancer is one hundred times worse.

We saw Dr. C at Moffitt today. Wow. Was Heidi ever correct. I'm so glad we listened to Dr. K about going. He asked so many questions to try and get a better understanding. Listened to my chest. Asked more questions, and then said, "I'm not sure what you have but I'm pretty sure it isn't lung cancer!" Hearing that from an oncologist lifted both of our spirits.

Dr. C said there were a battery of tests that he could run, but it didn't make any sense to him to do these tests before we got the results of the biopsy. MK and I loved his style and his ability to make a patient so glad to be in his hands—even if you don't need an oncologist.

Late that afternoon we got a call from Carrie, Dr. K's nurse. I shared what we had learned, and she was shocked that we hadn't gotten any results yet from the biopsy. She said, "Let me make a phone call or two – I'll call you back."

Thirty-one minutes later she called us back with the news: she had the results! All she would tell us is that the results were "better than we hoped." She asked if we could make it to Dr. K's office the next morning by 9:30.

Heck, with news like that I told MK that we could have made it to Dr. K's office in the next 10 minutes – even though it is a 20-minute drive.

Tonight, is another call with Doug and Liz. Can't wait to share this with them.

Then ... patience for 15 hours until we go to Dr. K's tomorrow morning.

Tuesday, December 13, 2022
Day 41

I really wasn't sure if I would sleep at all last night. We knew it was better news than we thought it would be, but we didn't know how good it was yet.

This was the 40th day since we got the diagnosis from the ER. I thought about the significance of forty in the Bible.

- Jesus spent 40 days in the desert wilderness before beginning his public ministry and was tempted by Satan all those days.
- Moses met with God on Mount Sinai for 40 days and 40 nights before he got the ten Commandments. He didn't eat bread or drink water during that time.
- The Prophet Elijah fasted for 40 days as he traveled until he reached Mt. Horeb, the mountain of God.
- Goliath threatened the Israelites for 40 days before David showed up with a sling.
- Jesus spent 40 days on earth after his resurrection before ascending into Heaven showing people, he was an alive and giving them proof.

Obviously my 40 days isn't biblical, but it is significant in our lives.

The news from Dr. K was better than we'd ever imagined: THERE IS NO CANCER! There was something weird in my lungs going on that mimicked cancer in CT scans. We'll deal with that but not today. This was a day of celebration. A day to let the prayer warriors know that their prayers have been heard and answered.

First, of course, we called the kids. We planned to have dinner with Jeff and Jae, or at least to go over and share a bottle of champagne with them. She has been right there through the process.

When we sent the email blast to the prayer warriors, we started getting phone calls. Family, friends, people that we didn't even know knew about this but were praying. I'm sure we will go through more stuff to find out what exactly is in my lungs. But today, celebrations start with prayers of thanksgiving to our Lord.

Wednesday, December 14, 2022

Day 42

Still thinking about the past 41 days.

I think when you worry about something for this long, when you mentally think about things but don't really share them with anyone, when you pray so hard for something and what happened yesterday happens—all you can do is give thanks to God.

Thursday, December 15, 2022

Day 43

When you face a challenge like this, be ready for all the appointments, calls, confirming messages, and everything you might get from doctors and hospitals. It is part of the process. That's all. Or, should I say, that was the first four processes for me.

One of the best calls we got was from Carrie, Dr. C's head nurse at Moffitt. She and Dr. C had just read the biopsy and discussed it. I had a chance to share the input from Dr. K. Dr. C thinks that I think I should start taking prednisone for the next 30 days – 4 pills per day. They also think I should get a bronchoscopy. Something else I'd never heard about before November 3rd. She will get this scheduled during January.

Hard to believe it is only 10 days until Christmas. My mind has been on so much other stuff. The only thing consistent has been our morning devotions.

Reading Matthew Kelly's *Holy Moments*, a gift from Dina and Mike Owens. Dina was the CEO when we joined Dwyer Group over 13 years ago. Also reading Terry Pluto's *Faith and You* Volume 2.

Another favorite writer is Max Lucado. He is very entertaining. What a terrific way to start each day with these great authors, daily devotions, and prayers.

I looked at my calendar and saw MK and I had an appointment with Dr. Trish next week. So glad Jae recommended her to us. So important for me to have a good primary care physician.

Took me back to my childhood and Dr. Perez. I remember my mom taking me to him when I was five. Saw him until I was twenty-six and moved to Ohio. I trusted Dr. Perez so much.

I remembered when Joan got pregnant. We were both first-year students in college. My life was set. I was going to spend a couple of years at junior college in Rockford, then at a state university, then teach in a Lutheran school where I could be a teacher and coach for basketball, football, and baseball for kids.

Yep, life was ready and about to change.

I still remember taking her urine specimen to Dr. Perez. He came in and told me that sometimes it is hard to tell with just a urine specimen. In our case, however, there was no doubt she was pregnant.

Joan and I got married May 4th—both of us were just eighteen. We had three kids by the time we were twenty-two. Life was on. I could never afford to go back to school and raise a family at the same time. I look back now, though, and realize that I'm not sure we could have afforded to raise a family with a parochial schoolteacher's salary.

Friday, December 16, 2022
Day 44

It takes a couple of days for reality to hit. I want to go out front of the house and yell, "I am cancer free."

I went back and forth with Carrie from Moffitt last night and got emails at 10:44 p.m. and again at 1:05 a.m. regarding my last CT scan taken at Trinity Hospital with the biopsy. She wanted to get a copy that so they could compare all the scans. So glad I came to Florida to do all these treatments.

The good news also opened all our travel plans for 2023, all the things that were tentative. One of those is an event in San Diego in March that MK will take Sarah and Jae to called "Secret Knock." Dina from Dwyer introduced us, and we enjoyed it so much. Invitation only. Now MK can share this special time with the girls.

The most exciting part of today is that MK's sister, Marti, and her husband, Steve, are coming over from Orlando for a couple of hours as she is out of the hospital. We hope to help her manage emotions as she faces her own biopsy with unknown results.

Saturday, December 17, 2022
Day 45

Even though the Florida weather is changing and colder, the joy in our hearts continues to grow.

I had a great phone call with four of my old high school mates last night. We served on a committee this year to plan our 50th high school reunion in Rockford, Illinois. We knew each other in high school but not well. In the eight months we worked putting this together, we became like brothers and sisters. Fifty years later. The reunion in September was amazing! We remembered seventy of our classmates who had died.

I outlived the age of my father and my brother when they died. I have great doctors, working with one of the best cancer centers in the country. Have an amazing wife, amazing kids, great grandkids. Yes, I've had issues. But it wasn't cancer.

Sunday, December 18, 2022

Day 46

I'm not good at taking medicine. At 68, I doubt that I've taken more than five vitamins in my life—and those were Flintstone vitamins when I was a kid.

I remember MK's parents' pill boxes" in their later years. They both had a seven-day pill holder with all their pills for the following week.

Here I am now taking what I used to take plus four prednisone tablets a day for 30 days. Two amoxicillin and clavulanate tablets per day per Dr. C for 10 days the size of horse pills, and three sodium tablets that Dr. K said I need to take for low sodium. Geez. Where are Mom and Dad's pill boxes?

Now I better understand why older people's conversations revolve around their doctors, medical appointments, and the pills they take.

Being movie buffs, we enjoy a variety of movies. Some are old like "It's a Wonderful Life" that we watch every Christmas season.

Today we watched "The Story of David" with Richard Gere. I've thought about this so much because Jesus was "of the house and lineage of David." One would think that David should be a saint. The movie did an excellent job of depicting David's sins. His mistakes as a father. As a husband. As the king. Yes, he committed adultery, killed tens of thousands, wasn't good or loyal to his first wife, and had a man killed so he could marry his wife. Great guy, eh? Yet, he was forgiven, and Christ was a descendant.

Reminds me that **everyone** on earth today can get forgiveness for whatever they have done. That God doesn't keep score. How blessed we all are.

Monday, December 19, 2022
Day 47

Today we looked forward to our yearly checkup with Dr. Trish. Such a free spirit and one of the most positive doctors we've ever seen. Being in her care has been wonderful.

Both MK and I are really in good health—at least we think we are. But we want to make sure we get all the blood tests necessary, check everything in the doctor's box, and make sure we are doing what we can. Dr. Trish recommends we start doing yoga to remain as flexible as can be. She does yoga on YouTube—even has an 83-year-old patient who teaches yoga—said she is the most flexible woman she has ever seen. Recommends this for anyone who is ageing.

We informed her of the different recommendations from Dr. K, our pulmonologist, as well as Dr. C from Moffitt Cancer Center. She fully agreed with both recommendations as well as the treatments and prescription each recommended.

What a terrific way to start our day!

At 7 p.m. on Monday nights we continue to meet with Doug and Liz on Zoom. We love our prayer worriers! We've been blessed with quite a few, beginning when we joined Dwyer Group (Now Neighborly) in 2010. Dina was CEO back then and she led with a code of values. She would deny it

– but I'm a firm believer that the speed of the leader determines the rate of the pack. Always have. Always will.

Christmas is days away. The kids and grandkids are on their way. I don't have cancer. This might be the best Christmas of my life!

Tuesday, December 20, 2022
Day 48

Parenthood vs. Grandparenthood. Which is easier?

Might be the easiest question ever asked of a grandparent.

Andy and Sarah got married in October 2009. Both decided that when they had kids that Andy would stay home and raise them, and Sarah would be the breadwinner. Made perfect sense to me because Sarah was getting her master's in mechanical engineering and had an amazing job. In fact, she was hired as an intern at a great company and has been there ever since.

I was concerned, though, because of my three kids Andy was the most challenging. And now, he was to raise kids? I couldn't have been more wrong. Andy knew what it was going to take to be a good dad. In fact, he said he wanted to author a book: *How to be a Good Parent*. Chapter One: spend time with your kids. (Expletives deleted). Chapter Two: See chapter one. That's it!

As a grandparent I've had a chance to see their relationship from afar, then up close as we spend time with them. Their nontraditional roles work great for their family.

Today Andy and Sarah embarked on the 1200-mile drive from Ohio to Jae's house in Florida. MapQuest says it will take 17 hours. Not sure if that includes Atlanta or not. Whew.

My concerns for them as they drive in the ice, snow, rain and whatever are much deeper than my concerns about my issues. The boys are young. I'm 68. MK and I miss them so much—we can't wait until they get here. Even though MK was never blessed with her own kids, I think God saved her for mine and the grandkids.

Wednesday, December 21, 2022

Day 49

I'll take you back 55 years ago tonight. It was a Thursday night, my last day of school before Christmas break. We had a grade basketball game at Nashold School in Rockford. We lost a close one then headed home. Dad didn't feel good after the dinner Mom brought him, but he thought it was just indigestion.

I remember my dad lying down and I asked him if he thought he'd stay home the next day. I was hoping so as he was my best friend. Then, I went to bed.

Mom called up to the room saying we needed to put the car in the garage because she didn't want to leave it outside with snow coming.

I got dressed and went out with her to do it. When we came in, we walked into the room where Dad was and there he was—on the floor. He had fallen and hit his head on the corner of the desk. We didn't realize then, but he had already died of a heart attack.

Mom called the ambulance and Dad's best friend, his boss. His friend immediately came over to take us to the hospital where we found, officially, that he didn't survive. My best friend was dead. Theodore William Liston, August 23, 1913–December 21, 1967.

For years I hated this anniversary. But, with kids and maturity, I've learned to focus on the kids instead of myself.

Puts everything into perspective. I've lived fourteen more years than my dad had a chance to live. I am so blessed, regardless of what issues may be in my lungs or not.

Thursday, December 22, 2022
Day 50

Moffitt Cancer Center stays on top of everything. Today they let me know that I'm going to have a Zoom call on January 4th with the doctor and anesthesiologist who will do the bronchoscopy on January 23rd.

This is a day that we look forward to each year: The Annual Golf Outing with Greg and his family. Greg's three kids are like nephews and a niece to me. My kids are the same to them.

Each year we meet at a par-three course in Tampa. Two-person teams. Scramble. The rule is that you can't play with your spouse on either nine. We really don't keep score—at least not officially—but some serious golfers may try and beat the others.

An important dynamic about the relationship that Greg and I have is that we are opposites in so many ways. Politics. Athletic ability. Approach to many different things. We have never, and I mean not since we were both able to vote, filled out a presidential ballot the same way. Yet, our friendship couldn't be better. It is a lesson for people in America. There are two points of view, sometimes vastly different points of view, and it doesn't matter.

Friday, December 23, 2022
Day 51

The weather was perfect when the family got here on the 21st, but a cold front is going through the entire country. What was eighty last week at our house will be 44 today. 45 tomorrow. Back up to seventy by the middle of next week.

The sad part is not what is happening to us but what is happening across the country. Over 2,700 flight cancellations. We've traveled on Christmas day and the excitement of seeing family is so cool. So many people may not get to share it this year.

Jae hosts a themed party over the Christmas season when the family is here. They invite a dozen friends to join, and it is always an outstanding time.

This is one advantage of having kids young. You aren't a great parent then . . . but can be a great parent now and be highly active with grandkids. Not sure which is better.

Saturday, December 24, 2022
Day 52

One of the wisest decisions that my kids' mom, Joan, and I made after our divorce almost 40 years ago was to stay close. She remarried, I remarried, and we remember that we were too young to get married in the first place. The result has been that the kids include us, together, whenever they can. We have gone to her place on many occasions. She lives just ten miles from us now up North.

She and husband Dale come to Florida, too, for Christmas at Jae's. And it is simply one family, not two different families.

Our favorite Christmas Eve event is the church service, especially when the lights go out, candles are lit and the congregation sings "Silent Night." Starts the celebration of the birth of our Lord!

Sunday, December 25, 2022

Day 53

It is nice when you are retired for Christmas to land on a Sunday. When I wasn't retired, I just looked for an extra day off (although I understand the 26th is a holiday as is January 2nd).

Most people read Luke 2 from the Bible on Christmas. I don't know many, though, who read Luke 1:

> *This is how the birth of Jesus the Messiah came about: His mother Mary was pledged to be married to Joseph, but before they came together, she was found to be pregnant through the Holy Spirit.*
> *Because Joseph, her husband, was faithful to the law, and yet did not want to expose her to public disgrace, he had in mind to divorce her quietly. But after he had considered this, an angel of the Lord appeared to him in a dream and said, "Joseph, son of David, do not be afraid to take Mary home as your wife, because what is conceived in her is from the Holy Spirit.*
> *She will give birth to a son, and you are to give him the name Jesus, because he will save his people from their sins." All this took place to fulfill what the Lord had said through the prophet: "The virgin will conceive and give birth to a son, and they will call him Immanuel" (which means "God with us"). When Joseph woke up, he did what the angel of the Lord had commanded him and took Mary home as his wife. But he did not consummate their marriage until she gave birth to a son. And he gave him the name Jesus.*

We know that Mary was young, 14 or 15, but we don't know how old Joseph was. Experts say he was much older than Mary. Who knows? But we do know that Joseph was a God-fearing man who was respected.

But I think about this. Have you ever had an angel appear to you in person or in a dream? I can't imagine that happening. Then waking up and knowing exactly what you had to do. Talk about having faith! This is the wonder of Christmas to me.

On the Santa side of Christmas, the magic is having kids around and seeing the excitement on their faces. We were at Jae's house by 7 a.m. with a bunch of bagels and cream cheese. All the adults didn't get up and ready until 9. Never like that at my house when my three were kids. We got up when they got up-although we had to tell them one year that 3 a.m. was just too early.

I love Christmas!

Monday, December 26, 2022

Day 54

I'm just so happy the biopsy came back the way it did before Christmas and before everyone came down to Jae's for Christmas. There is excitement in that house all day, and night, long.

Today I took Noah and Isaiah to the movies to see "Puss N' Boots – The Last Wish," then to lunch at Wendy's. As a parent I wouldn't have purchased the 55-gallon sized buttered popcorn. As a grandparent, why not?

What I did forget is how absent-minded kids can be. We realized after we had lunch that Isaiah had left his coat at the movie theater.

As a dad I would have been upset. Now, a different person. It didn't take long to go back to the movie theater and get the coat, which thankfully was still there.

Tuesday, December 27, 2022

Day 55

Parents will always worry about their kids, especially when making a 1200-mile drive straight through. Andy, Sarah, and the boys were making that drive home today, and we prayed for little or no snow on the road as they headed North.

We will miss the kids so much until we head back up in May or so. We are now missing basketball games for each of them, missed a couple football games, and we'll see what we will miss in the spring.

It has been wonderful to be able to step away from doctors and hospitals for a week or two during the holidays. I'm taking my medicine as prescribed.

Wednesday, December 28, 2022

Day 56

I woke up reflecting on a story I recently heard.

A man fell into a 10-foot hole and started yelling for help. The first person who heard him was a doctor. The doc wrote a prescription and dropped it down the hole. The next person who walked by was a minister. He wrote out a prayer and dropped it down the hole. The third person was the man's best friend. When he heard his friend yelling, he jumped down in the hole. When questioned why he jumped down into the hole the friend replied, "I've been in this hole myself, but I know how to get out."

How many times have we all been in a hole, not having any idea of how to get out? That funk . . . that depression. All we need is someone to grab us by the hand and assure us that they have been there before, and they can show us how to get out.

Mentors can do this. Biographies about the most successful people teach us that to get where they are today, these people went through so many trials and challenges. When I look back at my own life, some of the best memories are when I overcame adversity when I thought there was no way I could overcome those challenges.

If someone comes to me and asks for help to overcome something like what I have already faced, I'm glad to help them.

Thursday, December 29, 2022
Day 57

Anticipation.

My mind, first thing this morning was on the next month. CT scan, bronchoscopy, blood test, follow-up calls with good/sad news. Stupid. Why worry? There is nothing I can do about it. Remember, Mark, you *don't* have cancer!

One of the gifts in my Christmas stocking was a wristband from a company named Zox. They make inspirational wristbands along with other things. When I opened mine, it read "God's Plan." There is that whack on the side of my head I needed. I'll wear this wristband every day if it lasts. Along with this, l wear a "God is Good All the Time" wristband that I've worn since Doug was in the hospital after his bike accident.

Choices.

When I met Mary Kay, she told me her favorite word was "choices" because our entire life is about making choices. Anytime I screwed up in life it was simply because I made a bad choice. Friends, women, jobs, investments, everything. One of our favorite people to listen to on the radio is Dr. Laura. (drlaura.com). She ends every segment of her four-hour show with "Now go do the right thing."

Same stuff, right? Do the right thing . . . make good choices.

As we go into 2023, I hope and pray it is a year I make the best choices I ever have. If not, I know MK will help guide me . . . gently!

Friday, December 30, 2022
Day 58

I think about how to keep getting better in life.

First, do you want to get better in the various parts of your life? Financially, physically, emotionally, as a partner, as an employer or employee, in golf, and the list can go on in every area. One thing's for sure: if you want to get better, you can't do the same things in 2023 that you did in 2022.

In business one of the messages, we listened to every morning is Darren Hardy's "Darren Daily. It is free and focuses on life and business.

Today's Darren's morning message is worth remembering.

It is a story written by a cab driver who picked up a very elderly lady with a small suitcase and a box full of pictures. When they got into the cab, she explained that she was going to hospice.

She asked the cab driver if they could drive by a couple of places. At that point he turned off the meter and told her he would take her anywhere she wanted to go. They went to several spots in town that brought back memories for her. Eventually she told him she was tired and ready to go to hospice. She tried to pay him for the drive, but he refused. He realized that this was the last trip she would ever take in her life, and he was privileged to take her on that trip.

He didn't pick up anyone else that day and he drove around thinking about what had just happened. He also thought how fortunate it was for her that she had a cab driver who was kind to her.

The lesson from the story: People will not always remember what you do or what you say, but they will always remember how you made them feel.

What a fantastic way to end the year—especially as I think about all those people who have cancer or other life-threatening issues as they make their final journey.

Saturday, December 31, 2022
Day 59

Looking back on the past year, it has been a year of excitement, travel, cheering on kids' sports . . . then two challenging months that we couldn't have predicted. We may not know the reasons for the challenges over the past 59 days. But someday, someone will know. We look forward to a New Year with our lives in His hands.

God is in control in our life in 2023 just like He was this year. Life is good, life will be good next year, and we give all glory to Him!

Sunday, January 1, 2023
Day 60

Happy New Year! It is wonderful living by Jae and Jeff and being able to celebrate events like New Year's Eve together. Only a two-mile drive home, on side roads, and we can watch closely for any drunk drivers who are out.

One of our favorite exercises each year. MK and I review our goals for the previous year and put together new ones for the upcoming year. We started this about a decade ago and it is amazing how it changed our lives.

We base this exercise on Matthew Kelly's book *Dream Manager*. Amazing what one can accomplish when they set the sails for their own life. Kelly's book has a template to set your goals in various areas of your life. This is necessary for everyone as far as I'm concerned. Your life's goals change from year to year in so many ways. Plus, it is wonderful to see all you accomplished the previous year.

It sure beats just having New Year's resolutions. You know, the ones you break by the end of January!

Monday, January 2, 2023

Day 61

Two months ago, it was November 3rd—the day this all started. Amazing how the mind works toward the negative. Thinking about the Zoom calls already. It is because they will be talking about bronchoscopy, which I had never heard about until a couple of weeks ago. Wednesday Zoom call is simply with the doctor, I think, who is going to do this on the 23rd. Worrying for nothing.

We hate taking down Christmas decorations. We love leaving them up and the lights on 24/7. In front of the Nativity creche was a candle, the fake kind we all use today, that kept this lit up. Our creche was handmade in Germany and we bought it when we went to Oberammergau last year for their once-every-ten-years Passion Play.

Today we took down all outside lights, too. Nothing looks like Christmas, and it is sad.

Tuesday, January 3, 2023
Day 62

Over the years one of the subjects, I found myself preaching about, but only to those who weren't good at it, was customer focus. In my work life I used to take calls from upset consumers around the country who didn't get satisfaction because their local franchisee didn't *fill-in-the-blank*.

I wish I could have talked about Moffitt Cancer Center then. True to form they called me today to make sure I was ready for tomorrow's two Zoom calls. Besides double checking my birth date and current medications, the center had previously sent me the link to click on for each of the two meetings. The person calling had me go to that link, click on it, then did a 30-second call with me making sure it would work perfectly for me as well as the doctors tomorrow. Wow.

As I was jumping into bed last night, I turned on Monday Night Football and saw what had happened in the past 45 minutes with Damar Hamlin of the Buffalo Bills. He made a tackle and suddenly went into cardiac arrest.

Immediately after the game stopped, medical personnel rushed on the field to save his life, followed by an ambulance that quickly sped to the hospital. The players on both teams took a knee to pray. Tears streamed from players on both teams. Officials cancelled the rest of the game.

I hate to admit this but I'm a political being who, too easily, can find fault in our legislators. Ok, I can do it daily. I'm also terribly upset about the shootings in America—not just in schools—and how we are tying policeman's hands when they are just trying to serve and protect (their motto). MK's Godson is a police officer, and her brother-in-law is a retired police officer. We realize what they walk into every day. I don't know many others who would do the same.

Anyhow, I'm jolted into reality that regardless of how some fight "Under God" in the Pledge, when trouble comes the first thing so many do is pray. Wow. There is hope for us yet.

Then I learned about Damar Hamlin's toy drive for kids. $2,500 was raised over the past two years. Within 17 hours after the injury an additional $4.4 million was raised. Another wow.

When I see people reacting like they did in the past 18 hours I feel emotionally recharged. Yay for America. Yay for God-loving, giving people who know the first thing to do is pray, then help. We saw this on 9/11 in New York. As sad as that day was for America, the people in New York responded like none have ever before.

There is no question who is in charge. Just take one of the green bills out of your purse or your wallet and read the words "In God We Trust." Yes, He is in charge! What a terrific way for me, personally, to celebrate our grandson Joe's 16th birthday!

Wednesday, January 4, 2023
Day 63

Of course, I woke up thinking about the two Zoom calls. At 9:00 I got a call from the nurse practitioner who was making sure I was ready for a general anesthetic for the bronchoscopy. She had a cancellation and said we could get this in now versus 10:30. Perfect. This was the first time I heard the details of the procedure. It lasts about two hours, and they had one hundred questions on how I've tolerated general anesthesiology in the past. It has never been an issue.

A half-hour later I had a Zoom call with the doctor who will do the bronchoscopy. I learned then it will be the 24th – not the 23rd. She also went into detail about what she saw in the CT scans and what she hopes to see in the CT scan on the 12th. If all is clear she will cancel the bronchoscopy—wonderful! Then she'll recommend another CT scan in a couple of months. This is one of the reasons I love working with Moffitt.

She also said that if they do a bronchoscopy, they will do another biopsy on the worse looking mass based on what they see on the CT scan on the 12th. Perfect.

My takeaway from all of this is that it is so important to choose the right person—and I'm talking about the right spouse, right primary physician, right oncologist (should you need one).

If you own a business, you need the right attorney and right accountant. In every phase of your life, it is so important to know you've got the right people working with you! We had the right people as our prayer warriors!

It is so important, if one is going to make any changes in one's life at the beginning of a new year, that they start out right away.

Thursday, January 5, 2023
Day 64

Wondering today as I woke up if I will feel different once I am done with the prednisone. I feel great! Want to continue this feeling, medicine free.

MK and I continue trying to walk each day at least 5,000 steps. We went for a few months not worrying about walking any specific number of steps at all. When I do interviews with the doctors for anything they ask about my workout regimen. It is nice to be able to give a satisfactory answer!

Friday, January 6, 2023
Day 65

I've enjoyed playing golf for many years—since my twenties. Along the way, though, life got it in the way.

What was so important in my twenties is so less important now that I can, and should, play. I have a set of clubs in Florida and in Ohio. And no excuse. Greg is in Florida and Andy and Noah are in Ohio. Plus, MK will play a scramble round anytime we want.

Greg and I are both retired now, so costs are important to us. Greg paid for a special Florida golf card this year, so he gets great rates. I don't. He invited me to play today about an hour north of us at a course that he has played but I never have.

Greg is still playing softball with some guys over seventy. Amazing. He was a stud at softball in our twenties.

On the 17th hole Greg got his first hole in one. 126 yards, over water on a beautiful hole with a nine iron. Hugely elevated tee box— must have been 120 feet higher than the green. Think twelve stories higher.

He is sixty-six and looking at both knee replacements in the next two months. (Guess when you are a stud your body parts wear out sooner. I'm not worried.)

What holds me back from playing with Greg is that I'm so cheap. Except for DIRTBAG.

At our church in Waco, I joined a Men's Fraternity, a three-year course. We'd meet at 6:30 a.m. once a week so we could be in our offices before 8 a.m. to start our workdays. A different guy hosted breakfast each week.

Dr. Robert Lewis created Men's Fraternity. The first three years has three video series and workbooks entitled The Quest for Authentic Manhood, Winning at Work & Home, and The Great Adventure. The course was designed to help men come together and strengthen each other through weekly sessions that combine biblical teaching and small-group interaction.

These time-tested resources have been used all over the world to equip men to make their pursuit of noble manhood a lifelong priority. Church leaders and lay members are using the series to energize the men of their church and to connect with men in the community. Individuals have also used the series in their own personal pursuit of authentic manhood.

I had never been in a "men's only" group before but it was wonderful. I learned so much.

One of the key tips I took out of this was for fathers with adult sons: what are you doing each year with your sons?

Geez. Nothing. Wonderful job, Mark!

I thought about it, prayed about it, and decided eleven years ago to start a tradition. Both Andy's and Marcus's wives were pregnant, so we decided to do the first year in Ohio, within a couple of hours of both their homes. I flew Jae's husband in for the golf outing.

Eighteen to thirty-six holes on Thursday, thirty-six on Friday, thirty-six on Saturday, and eighteen on Sunday. I paid for lodging, food, and drinks. All I wanted that weekend was 15 minutes of time to talk to them about their lives and responsibilities. Something I wish I would have had someone to do for me.

We needed a name for the event. Evan Longoria of the Tampa Bay Rays graduated from Long Beach State. The name of the team there is the DIRTBAGS. And they sold DIRTBAG shirts, hats, and other merch.

It was now official: we had THE DIRTBAG OPEN. Andy is a serious golfer. The others, not so much, so we would scramble to try and beat Andy.

We went to a new location each year up until Covid. We've played in Ohio, Florida, Illinois, Wisconsin, Costa Rica, Myrtle Beach, and North Carolina, and we'll start the event again in 2023.

Over the years I invited Jerry's son, Tom, who is like a brother to my kids. Greg and his close friends, Pat, and Bob joined us. I don't pay for their golf but always cover Tom's, as he is like one of the kids.

This is an amazing event. Not because of golf. Not because of even the fifteen minutes with Dad. It is an amazing event because we are doing things as a large family of friends once a year. It is one of the highlights of the year.

Saturday, January 7, 2023

Day 66

The first Saturday of the month between September and March, our Florida clubhouse hosts a pancake breakfast. Only $3 for three pancakes, sausage, orange juice, and coffee.

Guys from the neighborhood volunteer to put it on. One of MK's and my commitments is getting to know more people in our neighborhood. I imagine there are 500+ houses/condominiums here. Nice clubhouse and pool. Not a golf community but there is a course a couple of miles away.

I love pancake breakfasts where guys all work together to put them on. Reminds me of what we did at our church in Waco on Easter. Same thing happened and it was so much fun.

MK checked on the details yesterday when she was at the clubhouse for Bible study. Someone told her I needed to be there by 6 a.m. and ask for Larry. I left the house about 5:30 and walked over—got there by 5:40—you know that Lombardi time thing that is stuck in my mind.

By 10 a.m. we served 173 people. We had twenty-five guys volunteering to help. Nice group of guys. Jeez, I'm getting older. This is a 55+ community. I think I look like one of the younger guys. I'm sure I'll still feel that way when I'm 75— at least I hope I do.

When I finished, I went over to the bocce court. MK was playing and I was able to join in. Play better bocce than golf. Still thinking about Greg's hole-in-one, though.

Sunday, January 8, 2023

Day 67

I'm passionate when it comes to church-shopping. In the past 30 years I've lived in Ohio, Illinois, Wisconsin, Florida, Texas, Michigan, and now back in Ohio and Florida again. I love being inspired on Sunday mornings. It has nothing to do with the size of the church; it has to do with the heart of the pastor. And their message each week.

We miss Pastor Rita here. I know it won't be long until we change Florida churches.

Reminded, again, today of how good Moffitt is. Already got a survey from them about the Zoom call I had this week. This is going to be a busy week. Blood test for us both on Wednesday and the CT scan on Thursday afternoon.

Once I realized the date I thought back three years to January 8, 2019—the date Mary Kay's Mom died. Ruth Shields had more lives than a cat! We said goodbye to her before surgery several times. She had a stroke when she was younger than we are today. Puts things in perspective. When I first knew her, she was going into surgery to put a bovine valve in her heart.

She invited MK and I to go into the room before that surgery when she was talking to the nurse who asked her if she'd ever had a hysterectomy. She replied, "Yes, honey, they took out the cradle but left the playpen." What a woman.

Dad was at sea for up to six months at a time, leaving Mom with six kids—a son and five daughters, of whom MK was the oldest girl. Mom had to work the all-night shift as a nurse delivering babies, then come home and sleep while the kids were at school.

In her spare time, she built a Heathkit color TV and a Heathkit organ, and she made sure all six kids were at Mass on Sunday morning. Her rule was that if they made it in time for the Gospel reading, they were on time.

In later years she got ovarian cancer that metastasized into other cancers. Eventually she and Dad moved into assisted living. MK was there when she passed at 89.

I'll never forget the funeral. By this time Dad was ninety and aging quickly— using a walker. The priest asked the kids to line up by age and to have Dad carry the urn with the ashes to the altar. The priest insisted that just as they walked down from the alter after becoming husband and wife, Dad should walk up to the altar, one more time, to give her to God. Not a dry eye in the church.

When I met her, she had this love of life and a laugh that few people have but everyone yearns for. Our senses of humor matched perfectly. She just called me "honey." She loved all my kids like I did.

Mom and Dad came to Jae's 40th birthday party, what looked more like a carnival than a birthday party. Dad even went into the dunk tank. Jae has always had the best parties!

Jae also went on the cruise for Mom and Dad's 60th anniversary celebration. One night on stage there was a "Newlywed Game." Mom and Dad won that hands-down.

As Mom went into one of her surgeries, Jae was there to give everyone a moustache. Mom wore hers as she went into surgery. What a gift to be Mom's son-in-law.

I've been so blessed.

Monday and Tuesday, January 9-10, 2023

Days 68 & 69

The medicines are running out. The sodium pills are gone as of today. The prednisone will be gone after tomorrow morning.

Our blood tests are tomorrow. Thursday is the CT scan. Let's pray all goes well with both and that the medical stuff is completed this week.

Wednesday, January 11, 2023
Day 70

Blood test day. The one test neither of us had to study for or be concerned about.

Thought about mentors today while MK was getting her blood test.

We have all had mentors who got us where we are today, haven't we?

MK and I didn't want to move to Waco. We didn't know anyone in Waco except for a couple of the people we would work with, and we didn't know them well. I wasn't a Cowboys fan or a Rangers fan. I didn't own a cowboy hat. Nor cowboy boots. Nor a cowboy belt buckle. But here we were in the city known for the Branch Davidians.

We knew of the CEO, Dina Dwyer-Owens from the IFA, and that was reason enough to leave Florida for opportunities presented both of us at Dwyer Group (now Neighborly).

MK and I learned so much from Dina over the 10 years before retirement. Similarly, we had learned so much from Joe Bourdow, the President of Valpak when we were there. Both were great mentors.

Jae and I joined Dina on a mission trip to Haiti with Mission Waco. MK and I went to Lead Like Jesus with Dina and her husband, Mike, where we met and learned from Ken Blanchard, the well-known author of so many books including *One Minute Manager*. We traveled with Dina and Mike for work, and we traveled with them and other executives on personal vacations. Dina also introduced us to The Secret Knock, where MK is taking Jae and Sarah to an event in March of 2023.

Thursday, January 12, 2023

Day 71

CT scan day.

Friday, January 13, 2023

Day 72

I've always liked Friday the 13th. Probably because so many others think it is unlucky! Not me, though.

All my prescription medicine from Dr. K and Dr. C. has been taken. All the tests are done. Waiting now to see the CT scan results so the doctors at Moffitt can decide if I need to have a bronchoscopy on the 23rd. Dr. K appointment next week. The process is moving along.

Had to get a copy of the CT scan so I could take it to Dr. K for Tuesday's appointment. Dr. K is not part of the Moffitt system, so I needed to drive to Moffitt—about a 45-minute drive with no traffic. So, at least a two-hour trip. As always, I listened to something on the radio while my thoughts wandered.

I spent seven years in the finance business. So many divorce issues and bankruptcy issues were simply a result of not paying attention. One spouse would blame the other for the monies they were spending. Usually, it wasn't discovered until the credit card bills came in or when the bank statement arrived.

And, I was guilty, too, of not working on what we were going to spend with my spouse.

MK and I use just two credit cards: one for travel and one for the rest. But we always—and I mean always—pay the balance in full at the end of a month. You don't ever pay interest and you'll never get yourself in trouble.

Saturday and Sunday, January
14-15, 2023

Days 73 & 74

The church we attended last week has a traditional service with the songs I learned as a kid, and a contemporary service with the songs that we listen to on the radio. There is also a Saturday night service like the 10 a.m. service on Sunday. We loved the contemporary service.

Reminds me of University Lutheran Chapel, the church we attended in Ann Arbor, on the campus of the University of Michigan. Great pastor, great music, wonderful experience— every week.

Monday, January 16, 2023

Day 75

Looked out the picture window in the living room that faces the lake directly behind the house. Beautiful morning. A heavy mist over the lake. I saw four deer walking directly behind the house and in front of the lake. Soon the sun will come out and the mist will disappear. The deer will head into the woods, and I'll be amazed once again by the wonders that God created on earth—and where we are blessed to live.

Tuesday, January 17, 2023

Day 76

The rainbow at the end of the storm!

Met briefly with Dr. K., who was disappointed that we just had the scan and not a written report.

Dr. T called later that day, and what a call! The CT scan came back great. Our doctor who was going to do the bronchoscopy had wonderful news. She said I don't need a bronchoscopy. The prednisone and the antibiotic were doing their jobs.

Appears that the masses are shrinking. Not only wasn't there any cancer, but I didn't even have the organizing pneumonia or need any additional medicines other than what I've been taking.

I'll still meet with Dr. K next month, and Dr. T next month . . . then have another CT scan sometime in April. But now it is simply making sure all is working well in the lungs.

God is good. Prayer really works. The Prayer Warrior team was and is amazing.

This will be my final daily update. From here I'll focus on others' stories for the rest of the book. They are amazing—mine was simply 76 days of learning and sharing!

We believe my story was a miracle. From lung cancer, to lymphoma, to pneumonia, to nothing—all in 40 days. What a life lesson we received in a truly brief period. We are so blessed.

Afterword

Amazing how God works!

As we started authoring this book, I was inspired. Inspired to help people understand the emotions they will go through when diagnosed with something that is very scary. A diagnosis that is on one's mind 24/7—although they try not to worry about it.

When I heard the twenty-six stories from various people, I became more inspired than ever. I could have never imagined what they went through. The pain. The fear. The hospital stays. Chemo and radiation. The words from the doctor.

Looking back, I never thought of squamous cell skin cancer as real cancer. Both MK and I have had a couple of those cut out, but that wasn't *real* cancer . . . or was it? When I interviewed Pam and heard that her father, a doctor, died of squamous cell, it reminded me to ask MK when our next appointment with our dermatologist would be.

Then I thought of all the other life-threatening diagnoses. I remembered the day about seven years ago the week before Christmas, the day that I outlived the age my father and brother were when they died of heart attacks. No warning for either of them. Just a massive heart attack.

I thought of my friend, Mark, who had prostate cancer and died from it. Same age as I was. I wear my goatee in honor of him. Before he died, he told me that the months before he died were the most inspirational of his life.

For those last few months, everything was different for Mark. He learned to appreciate the mornings. Sitting on the lanai every morning and just talking with his wife. He saw the beauty in flowers. The gracefulness of birds. Life was different. Life was inspirational. Too bad it took cancer to appreciate the life he had and didn't realize it.

I love old rock-and-roll. '60s and '70s music. No country music, of course. Not a fan. Then MK and I went to see Casting Crowns. Then, Newsboys. We the Kingdom. Sidewalk Prophets. King and Country. Danny Gokey. Mandisa. Matthew West. Now we listen to Christian music 95% of the time. At home. In the car. Inspirational music.

I wouldn't know how to exist without Jesus in my life. Fortunately, MK believes in the same things I do. We worship together. In my past I didn't always choose someone with the same beliefs. Those issues hurt our relationships.

There are so many religions and beliefs in the world today. I will never apologize for talking about and praising Jesus. I am confident that my parents are in Heaven. I'm confident that my brother is in Heaven. And I am confident that I will join them when God says it is time for me to come home to Him.

Recently in our morning devotions, MK and I read Hebrews 11 together. This is a chapter of the Bible I recommend all people read. It is about having faith. It is also a chapter that talks about the sins committed by famous people in Biblical times.

Moses. David. Samson. Rahab. Think about their mistakes: prostitution, murder, adultery. Doubting God. They were forgiven. So are we with all the mistakes we've made.

I don't know how anyone can read the Bible and think this is just a nice fiction story.

As you've read in this book, most stories are notable examples of people having faith!

We get smarter as we get older. We have more faith. Not always, though. Didn't happen to the smartest man who ever lived: Solomon! He got too overconfident. Amazing how ego comes into so much in our lives.

As I've mentioned, we did and will always have faith. I know we are forgiven for all the mistakes we have made.

I love instant replays in sports. What I dread is going to the pearly gates and having St. Peter tell me, "OK, Mark, let's look at some instant replays of all the sins you've made in your life!" We are blessed because God forgave us of all our sins, and He doesn't keep the replay of our sins. We won't have to watch the "worst of" playback.

Acts 16:31 makes it simple. "Believe on the Lord Jesus Christ, and you will be saved." Can it be that simple? Or Romans 10:9, "If thou shalt confess with thy mouth that the Lord Jesus, and shalt believe in thine heart that God has raised him from the dead, thou shalt be saved."

I'm fortunate that I didn't have cancer or any other life-threatening disease. I've had an amazing life. An amazing wife. Loving kids and grandkids are the joy of our lives.

But when it is time for me to join my parents, MK's parents, and her brother in Heaven, I'm ready!

I hope that every reader of this book finds Jesus as I did so many years ago. Bless my parents for helping me find Him. Bless MK's parents for helping her find Him. Life is so much better with Jesus in your life.

If you have been diagnosed with any life-threatening disease, whatever it is, I hope this book inspires you to understand that no disease must be truly life-ending. And if it is the end of your earthly life, make sure you live your life to the fullest.

The rest of your life can be better than you ever imagined. Your choice!

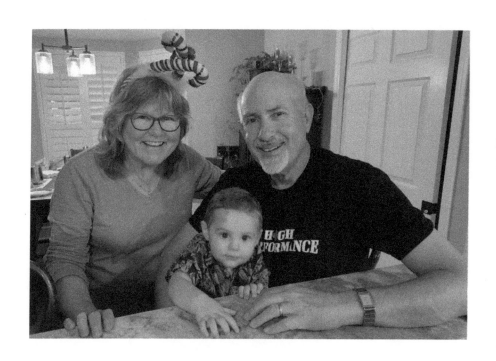

MK and Mark Liston with great-grandson

About the Authors

Mark and Mary Kay (MK) Liston are both retired franchise executives, retiring in late 2020 after a decade with Neighborly, formerly The Dwyer Group.

Mary Kay was the president of Molly Maid, the largest domestic brand of Neighborly, when she retired. Previously she was the president of Five Star Painting and the vice president of Operations at Mr. Appliance – both Neighborly companies.

She served on the International Franchise Association's Franchise Relations Committee.

After receiving her undergraduate from San Diego State, MK began her career in TV. After 11 years in broadcast television, Mary Kay launched her media sales career in cable TV. Starting as a commissioned sales rep in 1988, she quickly rose through the ranks to vice president of sales/general manager for Comcast Cable TV Los Angeles.

She oversaw four sales offices and centralized operations for a division with eighty-five associates producing over $30 million. She and her teams garnered awards for outstanding sales achievements.

While working for Comcast she went back to school and received her MBA from Pepperdine University.

Mark joined The Dwyer Group as vice president of operations for Glass Doctor in 2010, then became president of Glass Doctor in December of 2011. In all he has spent over 40 years in franchising.

One of the reasons for his success is working with the International Franchise Association (IFA), where he is still active today. He serves on the IFA Foundation and is past president of the Institute of Certified Franchise Executives. He also served on the IFA board of directors before retiring.

They met each other while working for Valpak in 2003. They got to know each other better beginning in 2005 and married in 2007.

They have twelve grandchildren and one great-grandson. They are blessed to be snowbirds and live nearby family all year round.

They worship in Rocky River, Ohio, at Good Soil Lutheran and in New Port Richey, Florida, at Trinity Lutheran.